Understanding Cosmetic Laser Surgery

Understanding Health and Sickness Series
Miriam Bloom, Ph.D.
General Editor

Understanding Cosmetic Laser Surgery

Robert Langdon, M.D.

University Press of Mississippi
Jackson

www.upress.state.ms.us

The University Press of Mississippi is a member of the Association of American University Presses.

Illustrations by Alan Estridge

12 11 10 09 08 07 06 05 04   4 3 2 1
∞
Library of Congress Cataloging-in-Publication Data
Langdon, Robert.
  Understanding cosmetic laser surgery / Robert Langdon.
    p.cm. — (Understanding health and sickness series)
  ISBN 1-57806-586-0 (cloth : alk. paper) — ISBN 1-57806-587-9
  (paper: alk. paper)
  1. Surgery, Plastic.   2. Lasers in surgery.   I. Title.   II. Series.
  RD119.L34 2004
  617.9'52—dc22   2003018609

British Library Cataloging-in-Publication Data available

Contents

Introduction

Perhaps you have been considering cosmetic laser surgery. A cosmetic surgical treatment is voluntary and not medically necessary. You must decide if such a treatment is right for you, and you will have to pay for the procedure with your own money. Health insurance does not cover cosmetic procedures. How do you know if a cosmetic laser procedure is worth it? How much improvement can you expect in your appearance? What are the advantages of a laser procedure compared to more traditional surgery? What is the down side of a given procedure? What are the risks, and how do these risks compare to those of alternative treatments? How do you know if a surgeon is qualified and can give you the best possible results?

The purpose of this book is to answer these and other questions about cosmetic laser surgery. Lasers have unique properties unlike any other surgical instruments. In fact, some cosmetic procedures would simply not be possible without a specialized laser. For decades many surgical procedures have been done using traditional instruments but can now be performed with lasers that offer significant advantages to the patient: advantages such as less bleeding or no bleeding at all ("bloodless surgery"), no scarring, much greater speed of treatment, much less pain of treatment so that little if any anesthesia is required, less postoperative swelling, and faster healing and recovery.

How can lasers offer so many advantages? One reason is that there are now many different lasers used for cosmetic purposes. Engineers and scientists have been hard at work developing new, specialized lasers for specific cosmetic applications. To understand why these machines work so well, one must have some understanding of human skin. Many lasers affect a precise component of the skin (usually the structure one hopes to eliminate) and that component only. The laser is designed for the express purpose of eliminating the unwanted skin component—for example, excessive facial blood vessels, pigmented birthmarks or age spots, aged or wrinkled skin, or sagging eyelid skin. However, lasers are not magical, and much of the perceived benefit of laser surgery is also due to the remarkable healing power of human skin.

Lasers are one of the most significant technological developments of the twentieth century. Lasers are machines that produce a pure and intense form of light that occurs naturally nowhere in the universe. The physical principles that make lasers possible were predicted early in the century along with other aspects of quantum theory. Albert Einstein conjectured about stimulated emission, the theory behind the design of lasers, in 1917. Researchers in the telecommunications industry understood the value that pure, intense light might have in conveying digital information and worked to develop a device based on those theories. By 1960, the first functioning laser had been developed. Within three years the new devices were already being used for medical applications. By the century's end, lasers had become the most ubiquitous practical application of quantum theory.

Many people encounter lasers nearly every day. Lasers are found in supermarket bar-code readers, CD-ROM and DVD-ROM computer drives, and CD and DVD audio and video entertainment systems. Fiberoptic cables carry most telephone and internet data in the form of myriad tiny flashes of laser light. High-energy industrial lasers are used to bore through steel. The unwavering straight line of a laser beam is used in transits by land surveyors and to make precise measurements in construction and road building.

Perhaps the most direct experience anyone can have with a laser is to be at the receiving end of a medical laser. The special properties of lasers have been used to great advantage in medicine and surgery. Many modern surgical procedures would be impossible without laser instrumentation. Surgical lasers produce specific effects that enable precise targeting of abnormal or unwanted tissue while sparing the "good" tissue. Treatments that were in the realm of fantasy a generation ago are now routine with specialized lasers: complete removal of a tattoo with no scarring or even any discernible change of the very skin in which the tattoo was implanted. Precise removal of thin layers of the cornea to change light refraction and correct eyesight exactly the way glasses or contact lenses would. Completely bloodless removal of delicate eyelid or facial skin. Rapid and minimally painful permanent destruction of unwanted hair follicles. These and many other surgical advances are only possible through the use of specialized lasers.

The majority of medical lasers have been developed for treating skin problems. Most of the new lasers are designed for cosmetic uses in the skin. A cosmetic application of a laser is very demanding. To be useful, the laser must be able to remove or destroy the unwanted skin component without damaging the other components. A cosmetic laser must be extremely precise and must have very specific effects. It is not acceptable to apply a "scorched-earth" approach and simply burn out a skin lesion in the same way that more primitive electrosurgery and cautery machines have been used for decades. Excessive damage of the skin resulting in a scar is not acceptable. In most cases the original skin problem looks better than a scar.

The successful development of useful cosmetic lasers has largely been the result of ingenious engineering. Special flashlamps and chemical switches have been used to devise pulsed lasers with very high power output over a very brief duration. Combined with the appropriate wavelength of laser energy, these pulsed lasers provide the needed precision and specificity to treat a wide variety of cosmetic skin problems. Wavelength (or color), one of the fundamental properties of light, largely determines what skin component will be affected by a laser. Different skin components, such as pigment, absorb certain wavelengths of light much more than other wavelengths. Cosmetic lasers are designed to exploit this specific absorption in order to produce a precise result (for example, removal of a specific skin pigment).

Many of the cosmetic skin lasers are so precise and noninvasive that they can be considered nonsurgical; these lasers are capable of removing only unwanted skin components without altering the overall structure of the skin. Unwanted blood vessels, pigmented lesions, tattoos, and even facial or body hair can be selectively removed, leaving behind completely normal-appearing skin. The special physical properties of lasers enable the remarkable precision and specific tissue effects that differentiate lasers from all other surgical instruments.

Skin is one of the few human tissues that can regenerate and be made young again. In the past few years, it has been the deployment of new surgical cosmetic lasers that has really captured people's imagination. Laser resurfacing performed by a skilled cosmetic laser surgeon can erase a generation of skin aging from the face. Although laser resurfacing is a superficial procedure (affecting only the topmost layers of skin), it can result in dramatic smoothing of wrinkles and tightening of facial skin, especially in patients with severe sun damage and wrinkling. Laser resurfacing alters the skin's structure and is thus a surgical technique. It replaces aged, wrinkled facial skin with a new layer of regenerated skin. Resurfacing lasers were developed using some of the same principles used in nonsurgical lasers, enabling precise ablation (removal) of thin layers of skin without imparting excessive heat to the skin, thus minimizing the risk of damage and scarring.

Another application of lasers to cosmetic surgery is the use of incisional or cutting lasers instead of scalpels. A major advantage of lasers over scalpels is that the laser can seal off blood vessels as it cuts through tissue. Bloodless surgery in many instances is safer than conventional surgery and results in faster healing with less swelling and bruising.

Knowledge of the structure and function of the skin is essential to understanding how and why lasers are useful tools for cosmetic improvement. Skin has several layers and is composed of cells and extracellular elements. The targets that cutaneous lasers are directed at vary from subcellular components such as melanosomes (pigment granules) to entire layers of skin. Because certain components of skin, as well as many types of lasers, possess precise and characteristic colors, preferential absorption of laser energy can selectively affect such specific elements as blood vessels or hair follicles or tattoo ink, leaving everything else undamaged. The laser is designed to affect only a specific colored target, or chromophore (chromo = color, phore = carrier). We will examine the major chromophores in the skin and the lasers that target them.

Many cosmetic problems of the skin are related to the aging process. What exactly happens to facial skin that makes people "look their age" (or maybe even older than their chronological age)? Many of the normal chromophores of the skin such as melanin (skin pigment) and hemoglobin (in red blood cells) become exaggerated and more prominent during the aging process and can be selectively removed with nonsurgical laser treatments. With aging the overall skin structure and texture is altered, especially in the more superficial skin layers (see chapter 2). Because superficial skin layers can regenerate, remarkable improvement in appearance can follow laser resurfacing. The real benefit of this treatment results from the skin's ability to renew itself. Under the right conditions, the entire face can be resurfaced and will heal without scarring.

We will explore the actual treatment process used for many cosmetic lasers. How is the laser energy confined to the target tissue? What is the end point that the surgeon is trying to achieve during the laser treatment? What is it like to be the patient? Does a certain laser treatment hurt enough to require anesthesia? What type of anesthesia is used and how is it applied? What is the healing process like? Understanding how lasers work to treat specific skin problems will remove much of the mystery surrounding cosmetic laser surgery.

Chapter 1 will explore the special physical properties of laser energy and the machines that produce this energy. Chapter 2 introduces the reader to the structure and function of human skin. Chapter 3 discusses the changes that occur with aging of the face and neck, including those in the skin and in deeper structures. In chapter 4 we will explore how specialized lasers can be used to improve cosmetic problems of the skin. Chapters 5 and 6 describe what the patient can expect from treatment with nonsurgical and surgical lasers. Chapter 7 discusses adjunctive cosmetic treatments and alternatives to cosmetic laser surgery. Finally, chapter 8 provides advice on how you can obtain the best possible results from cosmetic laser surgery.

Understanding Cosmetic Laser Surgery

1. What Are Lasers and How Do They Work?

For a better understanding of the special advantages of lasers in cosmetic surgery, we need to know what a laser is. How is laser energy produced? What are the properties of laser light that distinguish it from conventional light or other energy sources? Why are lasers uniquely suited to treat special skin problems of cosmetic concern to patients? Is a laser really that special, and why? The story of lasers begins over a hundred years ago.

A laser is an instrument that produces a special type of pure, high-energy, directed light. The theory that led to the invention of the laser in 1960 dates from the nineteenth century, when German physicist Max Planck proposed the quantum theory of light. Planck argued that energy was composed of discrete packets, or quanta, in the form of photons. The Danish physicist Neils Bohr expanded quantum theory to help explain the structure of atoms. In Bohr's theory the central nucleus of an atom is surrounded by orbiting electrons that are confined to specific energy states. A given electron can be "excited," or pushed into a higher energy state, if it absorbs external energy. For each chemical element, electrons can occupy only certain specific energy levels (fig. 1.1). Electrons can also release energy and thus move to a lower energy level. Excited electrons are inherently unstable and will spontaneously revert to lower energy levels, emitting a photon that contains the exact amount of energy that was absorbed when the electron was excited previously. This process is called "spontaneous emission" (fig. 1.2).

Electromagnetic energy is in the form of photons that vary widely in energy level. Photons are discrete particles but also have wavelike properties (light waves). The energy level of a photon is described by its wavelength, which varies inversely with its frequency. High-energy photons have high frequencies and short wavelengths.

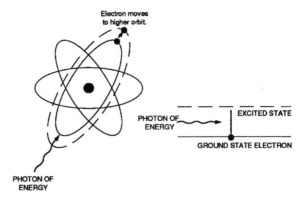

Fig. 1.1 Schematic diagram of an atom showing an orbiting electron in its ground state and in its excited state at a higher energy level.

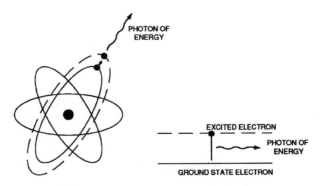

Fig. 1.2 Spontaneous emission.

Low energy photons have low frequencies and long wavelengths. The entire spectrum of electromagnetic energy ranges from very short ultraviolet (above the color violet) wavelengths to very long infrared (below the color red) wavelengths (fig. 1.3). Visible light is produced by photons with wavelengths lying between 400 nanometers (nm) and 700 nm. (A nanometer is one billionth of a meter; a meter is 39.4 inches.)

The visible part of the electromagnetic spectrum includes light of all colors that together appear white. A glass prism or raindrops

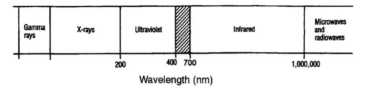

Fig. 1.3 The electromagnetic spectrum.

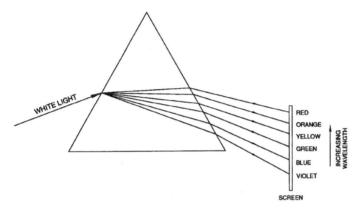

Fig. 1.4 A prism disperses white visible light into light of all colors.

in the sky will divide ordinary white visible light into its component fractions, producing a rainbow pattern (fig. 1.4). The longest visible wavelengths (and lowest frequencies) are red; every lower energy photon is in the infrared part of the spectrum. The shortest visible wavelengths (and highest frequencies) are violet; all higher energy photons are in the ultraviolet part of the electromagnetic spectrum.

The underlying principle of the laser phenomenon is stimulated emission, a theoretical concept that Albert Einstein devised in 1917. Einstein postulated that an atom that was already in an excited state (with an electron at an elevated energy level) and was then struck by a photon of like energy would be stimulated to release *two* photons as it returned to its ground (non-excited) state. He also conjectured that the two photons would have special properties, including identical energy levels (wavelengths) and perfect synchrony with each other,

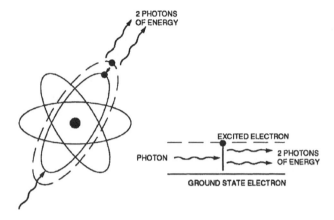

Fig. 1.5 Stimulated emission.

traveling in exactly the same direction (parallel) and with their wave-like properties in perfect phase (coherence) (fig. 1.5).

If a large number of like atoms are aggregated and then excited from an external energy source, so that many of their electrons assume higher energy states, many photons (all at the same wavelength) will be produced through spontaneous emission. If some of the photons strike other similar excited atoms, many of them will induce the process of stimulated emission, whereby a single excited atom now emits two identical photons. Under the right conditions a chain reaction ensues in which photon production is amplified. This process, and the apparatus that produces it, are both referred to as L.A.S.E.R. (Light Amplification by the Stimulated Emission of Radiation).

To harness laser energy, a laser apparatus is shaped like a long, narrow tube or cylinder. The cylinder has mirrors at either end so that photons are reflected back and forth and are constantly renewing the process of stimulated emission as they strike more of the excited atoms in the laser chamber. The mirrors also align the photons so that they are traveling parallel. One of the two mirrors is only partially silvered (reflective) so that it allows some transmission of the laser light. It is the transmitted light that becomes the laser beam (fig. 1.6).

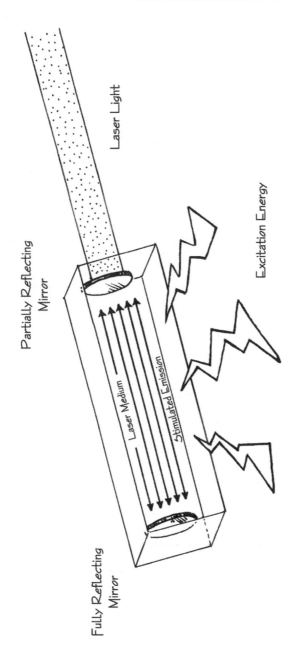

Fig. 1.6 Laser apparatus.

Special properties of laser light include monochromacity (all of the photons are at the same wavelength), collimation (all of the photons are traveling in parallel), and coherence (all of the light waves are in phase).

Monochromacity means being of one color (mono = one, chroma = color). The light of a laser beam is pure in that it is precisely of one wavelength. This purity is unique to laser light; all other light sources are of mixed wavelengths. Monochromacity enables great precision when a laser is used for medical or surgical purposes because components of human tissue preferentially absorb electromagnetic energy of specific wavelengths (see chapter 4).

Conventional light sources, such as an incandescent lightbulb, produce light of many different wavelengths that travels in all directions. An optical reflector can be designed to focus the light from a lightbulb into a directional beam, such as that used in a flashlight or an automobile headlight. The light waves are not truly parallel, however, and will soon diverge. In contrast, the collimated light waves from a laser diverge little over relatively great distances. An impressive demonstration of collimation of a laser beam was an experiment in which a laser beam originating on earth was pointed at the moon, which is 250,000 miles away. The area of the laser beam that struck the moon was only half a mile wide, thus the laser beam diverged by only one unit of distance for every 500,000 units that it traveled.

The third unique feature of laser light is coherence. Not only are all the light waves of exactly the same wavelength and running parallel to each other, but the crests and troughs of all of the waves are synchronous, or in phase (fig. 1.7). This highly ordered structure prevents individual photons from interfering with each other, enabling the laser beam to maintain its special properties of monochromacity, collimation and coherence over relatively great distances. A laser is thus a highly dependable, constant, and reproducible source of energy. Such an energy source is useful in meeting the exacting demands of cosmetic surgery: precise removal of unwanted tissue without affecting anything else.

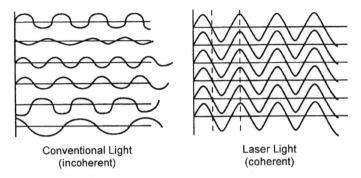

Conventional Light
(incoherent)

Laser Light
(coherent)

Fig. 1.7 Conventional light contains photons of many different wavelengths that are traveling out of phase with each other. Laser light is coherent: all photons are of exactly the same wavelength and are in perfect synchrony.

In the next chapter we will explore the structural features of human skin, in particular the physical properties of skin that enable the use of lasers to achieve safe and effective improvement in appearance.

2. The Skin

Normal skin is composed of a variety of cell types and extracellular materials. Significant changes in the skin's structure occur with aging. Both intrinsic skin pigments such as those present in birthmarks and exogenous pigments such as those present in tattoos can produce cosmetically objectionable skin lesions. Cosmetic lasers have been developed to treat many types of skin lesions by targeting the specific cellular or subcellular skin component that is responsible for the lesion.

Skin is the largest organ in the body by any measure: surface area, volume, or mass. It is much larger than its runner-up, the liver. Its most obvious and perhaps most important function is to provide a protective covering for the rest of the body and an interface with the environment. The skin is much more complex than it might seem at first glance. It has two major layers: the epidermis (literally, "on top of the dermis") and the dermis. As the name indicates, the epidermis is the outermost layer. It is composed of several distinct sublayers and one major cell type. There is a well-defined dermal-epidermal junction where the layers interface, below which lies the dermis. The dermis varies greatly in thickness in different parts of the body and provides nearly all the skin's structure, strength and mass. Below the dermis lies the fat layer, or subcutis (literally, "below the skin").

The major cell type in the epidermis is the keratinocyte (keratin = the predominant protein of the epidermis, cyte = cell). In most areas of the body the epidermis is only about as thick as a sheet of paper. On microscopic examination the keratinocytes are stacked on top of each other so that if the epidermis is cut in cross-section, it resembles a stone wall in which each cell is one of the stones (fig. 2.1). Keratinocytes are living cells that multiply rapidly in the lowermost or basal layer of the epidermis, then progressively flatten and change in composition as they die and are moved to the top layer (this change in keratinocyte structure is called

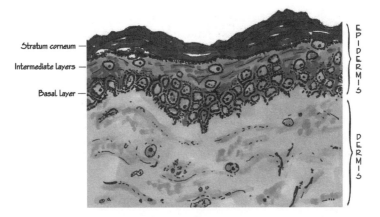

Stratum corneum —

Intermediate Layers —

Basal Layer —

EPIDERMIS

DERMIS

Fig. 2.1 Microscopic view of human epidermis and superficial dermis.

differentiation). As the epidermis constantly renews itself, the maturing keratinocytes migrate into more superficial layers of the epidermis. The topmost layer is called the stratum corneum and is the surface that you feel when you touch your skin. The stratum corneum is dry on the outside but also contains oils that make it waterproof. When you take a shower, none of the water gets inside you, but rather it beads up on the surface of the stratum corneum, much like rainwater on a waxed car. This waterproofing function is critically important and is one of the reasons that humans, who are composed mostly of water, are able to live in a dry, terrestrial environment. If this function is compromised (for example, by a severe burn), body fluids may be rapidly lost, threatening survival.

The lowermost epidermal layer is called the basal layer. The basal layer is moist and composed of a single layer of actively growing keratinocytes. The basal keratinocytes are among the most proliferative cells in the body and require large amounts of nutrition (which arrives through the blood vessels in the underlying dermis). The intermediate layers of the epidermis, the prickle cell layer and granular cell layer, are made of keratinocytes that are in the process of differentiating (fig. 2.1).

Another important cell type in the basal layer of the epidermis is the melanocyte, or pigment cell, whose primary function is to produce melanin, the skin's pigment. Melanin is a protein that absorbs ultraviolet (UV) light, protecting skin cells from UV damage. (People who are naturally dark skinned are genetically endowed with high levels of melanin.) UV exposure (such as from sunlight) stimulates melanocytes to produce more melanin. The melanin is packaged in tiny subcellular structures called melanosomes, which are transferred from melanocytes to keratinocytes where they reside. A tan is the skin's way of protecting itself from continued sun exposure. This protection is only partial, however, and the resultant sun damage is responsible for nearly all the changes that we associate with skin aging and even skin cancer (see "The Skin and Aging," below).

The dermis lies below the epidermis and comprises the bulk of the skin's structure and mass. Unlike the epidermis, which is mostly cellular, the dermis is mostly extracellular. Actual cells make up only a fraction of its mass; most of the dermis is made of proteins embedded in a watery tissue fluid. The dermis is both tough and elastic (shoe leather is made of cow dermis that has been treated with acid). It gives the skin both resilience and strength. Within the dermis are the blood vessels and nerves. Thus, if you get a cut, it will not bleed or hurt much unless the wound penetrates the dermis.

The blood vessels in the dermis are mostly capillaries and are normally not visible. Much of the skin's color that is not due to melanin is due to the red blood cells in the capillaries. (To appreciate this color contribution, try pressing hard with your thumb on your hand or forearm for two or three seconds, then release the pressure. This pressure squeezes the red blood cells from the dermal capillaries. The compressed spot will look much lighter for a couple of seconds until the blood flows back into the skin.) The redness of skin (especially the face) can vary widely depending on factors such as body temperature (for example, taking a hot shower) or emotional states (for example, blushing when embarrassed). The increased redness is due to dilation of capillaries in the dermis, permitting an increase of red blood cells (the red pigment within the cells is hemoglobin).

Other special structures in the dermis include hair follicles and sweat glands. These structures are composed of modified keratinocytes and can be thought of as invaginations of epidermal-type cells deep into the dermis; thus, they are literally epidermal appendages. The specialized keratinocytes that compose hair follicles differentiate into a hair shaft rather than into the stratum corneum that lies atop the epidermis. Many hair follicles, especially on the face, are associated with sebaceous (oil) glands, which are themselves composed of another type of modified keratinocyte (fig. 2.2). The lowermost extent of larger hair follicles may lie near the bottom of the dermis, and sometimes deeper still in the subcutaneous fat. Just as in the basal layer of the epidermis, there are melanocytes in the deeper part of the hair follicle. These melanocytes produce melanin, which is transferred to the keratinocytes within the developing hair shaft. The amount of melanin and even the type of melanin will determine the color and darkness of the hair. Some areas of skin contain great numbers of sweat glands (the underarm area, for example) or sebaceous glands (the oily areas of the face).

One common type of skin wound is an abrasive injury in which the epidermis has been completely removed and must then grow back. Hair follicles and glands within the dermis provide myriad sources from which epidermal cells may grow out to cover the wounded area. The modified epidermal cells from these glands and follicles are capable of reverting to typical epidermal keratinocytes as they proliferate and repopulate the resurfaced area. In this way, a new epidermis is regenerated and takes the place of the old epidermis. In facial laser resurfacing, the epidermis (and some of the superficial dermis) is purposely removed. Epidermal cells rapidly proliferate and migrate, covering an area as large as the entire face in about a week and a half.

The predominant cell type in the dermis is the fibroblast. Fibroblasts, which produce the dermal proteins, lie embedded in a protein-rich fluid and are separated from each other by at least several cell diameters. The major protein within the dermis is collagen, the most prevalent protein in the body. Collagen molecules are arranged into large, linear fibers (fig. 2.3). Water accounts for 70% of the mass of the dermis, whereas collagen constitutes 75% of the dry weight. After an injury, the fibroblasts sometimes produce excessive amounts of collagen during healing, resulting in a thick hypertrophic scar. The second most abundant dermal protein is

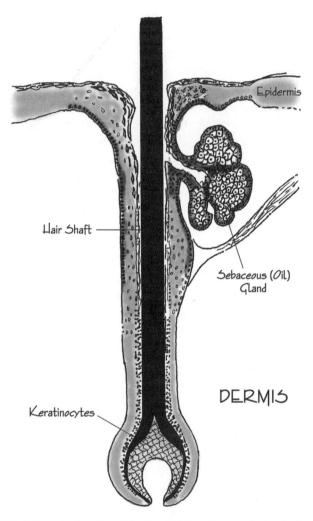

Fig. 2.2 Schematic drawing of the hair follicle with an associated sebaceous (oil) gland.

elastin, which aggregates into long fibers that can be stretched and will contract back to their original length, providing most of the skin's elastic properties. Elasticity is an important aspect of the skin's strength and resistance to shear forces and tearing. As we will see,

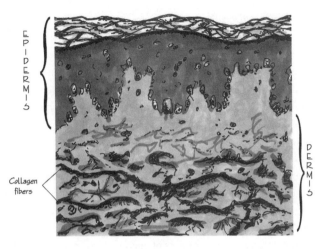

Fig. 2.3 Microscopic view of human skin.

much of the aging effects of sun damage on the dermis are caused by damage to elastin.

The Skin and Aging

Aging causes subtle structural and biochemical changes in the skin independently of environmental factors. The most obvious and characteristic changes, however, are largely the result of many years of sun exposure. How old one looks (especially in the face) is much more a function of how much sun damage he or she has suffered than it is of his or her chronological age. The sun produces a great deal of UV radiation, which is largely responsible for the skin damage. The damage ranges from an acute injury such as sunburn to the chronic structural changes that we associate with aging skin, including splotchy pigmentation (age spots) and wrinkles. Most skin cancers are attributable to UV damage to skin cells' genetic material: deoxyribonucleic acid (DNA). Protection from sun exposure is by far the most effective measure anyone can take to prevent aging of the skin as well as potentially serious health problems such as skin cancer. Even artificial sunlight (like that from indoor tanning) is a source of UV light that can significantly accelerate skin aging.

How does the sun damage the skin? What observable changes that we associate with aging can be attributed to sun exposure? To answer these questions, we can take a "top down" approach starting with the epidermis. In aged skin the epidermis is significantly thinner than it is in youthful skin. The number of cell layers actually diminishes, but the process of differentiation continues so that the skin surface is always covered by a waterproof stratum corneum. The epidermis never fails with old age, resulting in loss of its barrier function. Epidermal failure would be a life-threatening problem, because the person would literally dry up. In other words, nobody ever dies of "old skin" as they do when other life-sustaining organs such as the heart, liver, or lungs fail. A biopsy of aged skin from a chronically sun-exposed body area such as the face would demonstrate a thinner epidermis than would a biopsy from a rarely (if ever) exposed area such as the buttock. On the same person all of the structural changes of aging will be much more evident in skin from sun-exposed areas than in skin from sun-protected areas. In this type of "controlled experiment" the chronological age of skin from the two sites is identical. All of the additional microscopic signs of aging in sun-exposed skin are therefore manifestations of sun damage.

Aged epidermis may demonstrate rough and flaky spots that contain abnormal, precancerous keratinocytes. These spots are called solar keratoses (a keratosis is a thick patch of skin) because they are caused by chronic sun exposure. Severely sun-damaged skin may be rough due to the presence of myriad solar keratoses. These growths can eventually become cancerous.

Another characteristic of aged skin is uneven or splotchy pigmentation. A solar lentigo (age spot or liver spot; plural = lentigenes) is a flat, brown skin lesion with increased melanin in the epidermis. Sun exposure normally causes a tan to develop, in which pigment cells proliferate, producing increased melanin. After years of chronic sun exposure, some of the melanocytes in small areas (typically about half an inch wide) overproduce melanin on a permanent basis, even when the surrounding skin is not tanned.

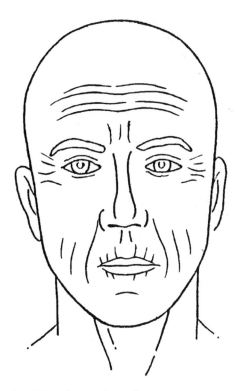

Fig. 2.4 Facial wrinkles characteristic of aging.

Profound structural changes in the dermis also occur with sun-induced aging. Whereas gradual thinning of the dermis is typical of aging in non-sun-exposed areas, thickening occurs in exposed areas. Greatly increased amounts of abnormal elastic fibers, many of which are fragmented or thickened, appear in the dermis. This phenomenon is termed solar elastosis. If severe, the excessive elastic tissue imparts a sallow, yellowish color to the skin. Another abnormality of the dermis is a change in its texture. The dermis becomes less resilient and stiffer. The most obvious manifestation of a less pliable dermis is facial wrinkles that develop where the skin is folded by the contraction of expressive muscles (fig. 2.4). For example, raising the eyebrows causes horizontal forehead wrinkles, frowning causes frown lines, squinting causes crow's feet wrinkles in the temple area, and pursing of the lips causes upper lip wrinkles. In youth, the resilient elastic dermis resists permanent wrinkle formation. With sun-induced damage, the stiffer inelastic dermis collapses into persistent wrinkles. Wrinkles, though evident on the skin surface, are actually a defect of the dermis. The epidermis is of equal thickness within and between wrinkles. It is the dermis that is thinner in the center of the trough of the wrinkle. The deepest wrinkles occur in facial areas with the greatest degree of solar elastosis, because the abnormally thickened dermis allows for even deeper wrinkles.

Overall skin laxity or looseness is another feature of sun-damaged facial skin. The primary force that appears to contribute to skin laxity is gravity. Over a lifetime, approximately two-thirds of which is spent in an upright position, gravity actually stretches facial skin, causing most anatomic features to droop. Gravity also gradually stretches the underlying fascia, the superficial connective tissue deep to the skin. The eyebrows sink, the nasolabial furrow (the deep groove that runs from the bottom of the nose to the corner of the mouth) deepens and the jowls (the lower cheek) drop below the jaw line. Facial skin becomes redundant; the excess skin accentuates the depth and severity of wrinkles.

Yet another sign of chronic sun damage is the dilation of facial blood vessels (these enlarged vessels are called telangiectases). Such enlarged vessels are especially common around the nose and in central facial areas. The vessels enlarge enough to become visible as discrete, linear blemishes. Although frequently referred to as "broken blood vessels," telangiectases are intact, functioning vessels. Chronic sun damage is the most common cause of facial telangiectases, but rosacea, a common skin disease that causes frequent flushing (blushing) reactions, can also cause them.

Smoking and the Skin

People who smoke heavily will undergo premature aging of facial skin that is additive to or synergistic with sun damage. The term "smoker's face" is used to describe the increased wrinkling and subtle orange-red discoloration that is common in smokers. Cigarette smoke includes toxins that cause constriction of dermal blood vessels via both systemic and topical (through the skin) exposure. Constricted blood vessels result in chronic poor oxygenation of the dermis. The structural changes in the skin may be partly the result of this decreased blood supply. Facial skin is directly exposed to heat from smoke; this thermal effect may contribute to damaging the skin.

Microscopic studies of smokers' facial skin have revealed increased elastic tissue in even greater quantities than that seen in people who have had comparable sun damage. This smoker's elastosis is analogous to solar elastosis and may account for much of the increased wrinkling and discoloration seen in smoker's face.

Exogenous Pigments

The pigments that contribute to the skin's normal color—melanin and hemoglobin—may be accentuated within benign skin growths such as moles and hemangiomas. A mole (the medical term is "nevus") is a collection of melanocyte-like cells, usually within the dermis. These nevus cells generally produce increased amounts of melanin, imparting a brown color to the lesion. (Nevi are discussed in greater detail in the section on Birthmarks, below.)

A hemangioma is a bright red bump that is composed of capillaries packed closely together. Although these lesions are raised above the skin surface, they are composed of dermal tissue (blood vessels) and are covered with normal epidermis. Hemangiomas are red simply because they contain so many red blood cells.

In certain abnormal or disease states, the skin may contain other pigments that produce unusual colors. Hemosiderin may make the skin appear brown or orange after a bruise or other injury heals, or after an injury that causes red blood cells to leak out of the capillaries (for example, a bruise). Macrophages, a type of white blood cell, are responsible for clearing out any substances that are normally not present in the dermis. Red blood cells that appear in the dermis after an injury die and then deteriorate; macrophages ingest the debris. Enzymes within the macrophages convert hemoglobin to hemosiderin, a protein that, like hemoglobin, contains iron. This substance may be present until the macrophages are able to physically remove it from the skin. The cleanup function of macrophages seems to be more efficient in areas of the body with good circulation (such as the face) than in areas with poor circulation (such as the lower leg or the feet). Hemosiderin is rarely encountered in the face but may persist for years in the ankle area.

Melanin may also get displaced as a result of an injury or inflammatory skin disease. Melanin is normally confined to the epidermis, but with an injury some of the melanin may drop down into the dermis. This displaced melanin will appear as a darker area of skin. A common cause of such post-inflammatory hyperpigmentation in the facial area is acne. Many people attribute this discoloration to scarring, but a true scar is a permanent alteration in the skin's texture (see Scars, below), with or without a change in skin color. Post-inflammatory hyperpigmentation is only a change in color and is not permanent; it will eventually disappear as macrophages remove it.

Hemosiderin and melanin are both endogenous protein products that appear naturally in the skin. There are also exogenous pigments that are the result of deposition into the skin of a manufactured or artificial material. An example of such material would be pigments that develop from topically applied or ingested drugs or medications. An intentional example of exogenous pigmentation would be a tattoo.

Certain drugs can accumulate in the skin directly or in an altered form due to changes in the drug molecule caused by sunlight or by the body's metabolism of the drug. Minocycline, an antibiotic used to treat acne, becomes chemically altered and forms slate gray deposits in the skin of some people. Amiadarone, a heart medication, causes a similar discoloration in nearly all patients who take it. Chlorpromazine, a drug used to treat mental illness, reacts with sunlight and causes discoloration of facial skin.

People have adorned their bodies with decorative tattoos since prehistoric times. Tattoos are produced by placing exogenous pigments into the dermis. Any pigment placed into the epidermis would quickly disappear by being carried away in the constant flow of keratinocytes migrating to the surface of the epidermis as they differentiate and finally flake off into the environment. Exogenous pigment material placed into the dermis will stay there, seemingly indefinitely. Tattoos are essentially permanent but may fade over many years as macrophages gradually remove those pigment particles that are small enough to be ingested.

The most common tattoo pigment, used throughout history and even in modern times, is carbon-based. Soot or charcoal from fires was used in ancient times as the carbon source and was implanted into the skin with small sharp objects such as bone chips. In more recent times the most commonly used black pigment has been India ink, which is composed of graphite (pure carbon) particles suspended in water. Tattoo ink is implanted into the dermis with needles. Because of the optical qualities of the skin, the black graphite particles frequently reflect a dark blue color to the viewer.

Other common pigments used for tattoos include cobalt (blue), cinnabar (red), and chromium (green). Recently, a variety of intense organic pigments have been used to produce tattoos with greater color saturation.

Birthmarks

Birthmarks are collections of cells or skin structures that are aggregated more densely than they are in normal skin. They are visible because they are composed of increased concentrations of the skin's visible pigments, hemoglobin or melanin. Less common birthmarks are normal in color but abnormal in texture because of increased thickness of the epidermis or dermis.

The most common vascular lesions present at birth or appearing in early childhood are "port wine stains" and hemangiomas. Port wine stains are generally smooth, flat red patches that occur most often on the face or neck and are composed of excessive dilated capillaries within the dermis. Variants, including larger blood vessels or hypertrophic (enlarged) dermal tissue, may result in a raised skin surface. In these lesions the flat port wine stain is combined with raised hemangioma elements. Without treatment, port wine stains generally persist throughout life. Over the years, untreated lesions may become darker or more elevated as the involved blood vessels increase in diameter.

Hemangiomas may be present at birth, but most develop in the first few weeks after birth. These dynamic lesions can enlarge over a period of a few weeks. Hemangiomas are composed of proliferative vascular elements including capillaries and supportive dermal tissue; they are soft, raised, and intensely red. If treated early by laser therapy, a small hemangioma may be prevented from growing into a much larger lesion.

Most hemangiomas will eventually shrink even without specific treatment, but untreated lesions usually transform into scar tissue with an abnormal texture or color. Most of the blood vessels will involute, but a few prominent ones may remain permanently.

Melanin is the other skin pigment present in excess in certain types of birthmarks. The term nevus is used by dermatologists to describe many birthmarks and acquired (appearing later in life) lesions. A nevus (plural = nevi) is composed of one or more epidermal or dermal cell types that are densely aggregated into a visible lesion. There are characteristic nevi composed of most different skin cell types (e.g., epidermal nevus, connective tissue nevus, melanocytic nevus).

The common mole or melanocytic nevus is by far the most prevalent pigmented lesion. A mole is usually brown due to the production of melanin by the nevus cells. Depending on the location of the nevus cells and their number, the mole may be flat, slightly raised, or dome shaped. The great majority of nevi are acquired (appear after birth), but some are congenital (present at birth). Whereas acquired nevi are usually small (less than a quarter inch in diameter), congenital nevi are generally larger and can even cover a significant percentage of the body surface.

All melanocytic nevi should be monitored closely for any changes in appearance. The modified melanocytes that compose these lesions can give rise to malignant melanoma, one of the deadliest forms of cancer. The key to combating melanoma is prevention, including behavior modification (avoiding excessive sun exposure, especially sunburn) and clinical surveillance. Dermatologists are highly trained in the recognition of abnormal nevi and subsequent biopsy (sampling) or surgical removal of these lesions. A computerized skin surface imaging system presently under development holds great promise to increase the efficiency and "throughput" of screening the entire skin surface for abnormal pigmented lesions.

Because of their increased size, congenital nevi pose a significantly greater risk of melanoma than do acquired nevi, and surgical removal of congenital nevi, if feasible, is frequently recommended. Very large lesions may be impossible to remove by conventional surgery; laser surgery may be the only option.

The Nevus of Ota (first described by M. Ota, a dermatologist in Japan) is a variant of congenital nevus that occurs (usually) on one side of the face. This lesion is relatively common in Asians and is a major cosmetic concern. The cells that make up the Nevus of Ota are located deep in the dermis. The lesion is generally flat and is usually dark blue due to the optical properties of light reflected from the skin.

Cafe-au-lait spots are common birthmarks composed of epidermal melanocytes that are increased in density as well as in activity (melanin production). These spots are a light brown or tan color and are usually one to two inches in diameter. They occur in up to 10% of the population. Cafe-au-lait spots are totally flat and smooth.

Scars

A scar is a permanent alteration in the skin's texture. Hypertrophic scars are thicker than the surrounding skin; atrophic scars are thinner (depressed). A scar is usually the result of an injury. Scars are an alteration of the connective tissue of the dermis. An injury that heals with the production of too much dermal collagen may result in a hypertrophic scar. If too little collagen is produced with healing, an atrophic scar may result.

The most common facial scars are caused by acne or chickenpox; most of those are atrophic. Acne scars may be classified by diameter and depth into three types. Type I scars are relatively small and superficial in depth. They are the most readily smoothed out by a resurfacing procedure such as that done by laser. Type II scars are small but relatively deep. These scars are best removed by excision and stitching the skin together or placing a small skin graft in the resultant defect. Type III scars are both wide and deep. The best way to improve this type of acne scar is to counteract the atrophy by making the skin thicker through a procedure such as tissue augmentation or subcision (see chapter 7).

Many posttraumatic scars differ in color from the surrounding skin. That, and their altered texture (hypertrophic or atrophic), contribute to their visibility. Within the first months or years following an injury, the scar may be redder than the surrounding skin due to dilated blood vessels, but the redness eventually fades. After that the scar may be more lightly pigmented because of a lack of melanocyte presence and/or function. Such hypopigmentation may be more difficult to improve than the textural abnormality of a scar. There is no consistently effective treatment for permanent hypopigmentation.

We have reviewed the special properties of lasers and those of human skin, including the effects of aging, smoking, and disease on the skin. Aging of the skin does not occur in isolation; subcutaneous tissues also undergo aging, especially in the face and neck. In the next chapter, we will discuss how aging occurs in different tissue levels and how cosmetic surgery can reverse the changes.

3. Facial Aging: More than Skin Deep

To better understand the role of cosmetic laser surgery in improving appearance, an appreciation of the anatomy of the face and neck and how the aging process affects these areas is needed. In most people the face and neck age concurrently because of structural overlap of these two areas. Aging occurs not only in the skin but at deeper levels independent of the skin, and they age for different reasons. Complete rejuvenation of the face and neck requires restoration of youthful features at all the levels at which aging occurs.

Anatomy of the Face and Neck

The face and neck share anatomic features at all structural levels. The skin is continuous over these areas but varies in its physical qualities as well as in its exposure to environmental insults. The skin varies in thickness in different areas of the face and is thinnest on the upper eyelids. (The epidermis is relatively constant in thickness; it is the depth of the dermis that varies from place to place.) Mid-facial skin tends to be thicker than average and contains abundant sebaceous glands.

The skin becomes thinner in the neck and contains fewer epidermal appendages such as sebaceous glands. The upper part of the neck is somewhat protected from sun exposure because it is in shadow below the jaw line and is therefore partly spared from the photo-aging that occurs in facial skin. In contrast, the lower and lateral areas of the neck suffer significant sun damage and photo-aging.

Just below the skin is the subcutaneous fat. In the face the fat layer is relatively thin; in non-obese people the jowls (lower cheeks) are the facial area most likely to develop an appreciable mass of fat. In the neck there is frequently a more substantial collection of subcutaneous fat near the midline below the chin. This area can be fatty even in otherwise slender people, usually the result of an inherited tendency (family trait).

Humans develop fat deposits in specific, characteristic sites. As people gain weight existing fat cells become larger (fat cells do not multiply) in these areas. Weight gain is common with aging, and in people who are even mildly obese the characteristic fat deposits become more pronounced. In more obese individuals, the middle neck area below the chin is one such characteristic fat deposit; others include the lower abdomen and upper outer thighs. Because weight gain is a feature of aging in most people, increased prominence of fat in the jowls and neck is a common manifestation of aging. Excessive fat in the neck can result in a "double chin."

Below the fat layer in both neck and face is a thin layer of connective tissue. In the neck, this layer is in the form of a thin, flat muscle called the platysma. There is a platysma muscle on each side of the neck. As the platysma crosses the jaw line and enters the lower cheek area, its muscle fibers change into collagen fibers or connective tissue; in the face this layer is described as fascia. The entire platysma/fascia layer is referred to as the "superficial musculoaponeurotic system" (SMAS). "Aponeurosis" is another term for fascia.

There are more than 30 facial muscles of expression, which account for the bulk of the face's soft tissue volume. These muscles enable animation and expression of emotion. Many facial muscles originate with an attachment to the skull and converge in the mouth area where they attach to the orbicularis oris, the round muscle that encircles the mouth.

Aging of the Face and Neck

The biggest challenge in cosmetic surgery is to reverse the signs of aging in the face and neck. Facial aging is a complex process that occurs at three different physical levels. The most superficial and visible level is the skin. The preponderance of sun damage is in the skin and is easily removed by surgical procedures such as laser resurfacing. With healing, entirely new layers of skin replace the sun-damaged skin, essentially reversing the aging process.

The second physical level of facial aging is just below the skin and subcutaneous fat in the connective tissue or fascia. The fascia is too deep to be affected by sun damage and ages through the effect of another physical force: gravity. There is no escaping gravity. Because we are constantly subjected to the force of gravity, and we spend most of our time in an upright position, after years we will all find that our fascia layers stretch and sag. Sagging of the lower face and neck produces jowls and a "turkey gobbler" neck. Near the midline of the neck the medial edges of the platysma muscles can become redundant, producing vertical ridges called "platysma bands." In the upper face, the forehead can drop and cause the position of the eyebrows to descend, contributing to the appearance of excessive upper eyelid skin. The solution to gravitational sagging of the fascial layers is surgical lifting such as facelift and forehead lift. In these procedures the fascia is directly pulled upward and tightened, and is anchored to unyielding structures such as skull bones. Prominent platysma bands can be eliminated by a procedure called platysma plication (also called platysmaplasty), in which the medial edges of left and right platysma muscles are stitched together so that they join in the midline of the neck. (For more on facelift and platysmaplasty, see chapter 7).

The third and deepest level at which facial aging occurs is the muscle and bone; with aging there is a loss of volume (atrophy) in both. Contoured surfaces that are convex (rounded) in youth (such as the cheeks) gradually lose volume and become flattened or even concave (indented). This volume loss is at first subtle but is noticeable even in individuals who have little sun damage or gravitational sagging, and is one of the unmistakable signs of aging. This atrophy is most pronounced in the mid-facial area and around the mouth. With increasing age the chin recedes and the lips become thinner. The cheeks can become sallow and indented. The exact cause of this deep level atrophy is unknown; it is probably determined by genetic tendencies. Certain disease states (e.g., AIDS) can greatly accelerate facial atrophy. The solution to atrophy is volume augmentation with natural materials (most useful is a patient's own fat tissue) or with synthetic implants (usually made of a plastic or silicon material). Fat augmentation has the advantage of being totally natural and works best when the fat cells are placed within the facial muscles. Fat augmentation is permanent and can restore volume deficits that result from atrophy of both muscle and bone. Alternatively, anatomical implants made of artificial materials can be placed in the chin or cheek areas. Implants are usually placed immediately above bone.

To restore youthfulness, all three levels (skin, fascia, and muscle) at which aging occurs must be addressed. Because aging occurs independently at each level and for different reasons, in certain individuals there may be a greater need to rejuvenate one level over the others. For example, in a patient who has suffered a great deal of sun damage, laser resurfacing, which rejuvenates the skin, would be the top priority. Those with less sun damage may benefit more from fascia tightening (e.g., facelift) or volume restoration (e.g., fat augmentation). In practice, most patients benefit from rejuvenation procedures at all three levels but can expect the greatest overall improvement from the procedure that they need the most.

In the next chapter we will learn about some of the actual cosmetic lasers that are commonly used to improve the skin's appearance, including why and how these machines work.

4. Lasers Used to Improve the Skin's Appearance

In this chapter I discuss the elements within the skin (chromophores) that absorb laser energy as well as the guiding principle behind all cutaneous cosmetic laser treatment (selective photothermolysis). I will recount the history of the use of lasers to improve the skin's appearance. This use significantly predated our understanding of both chromophores and selective photothermolysis.

The skin is the most accessible organ of the human body and is particularly well suited to treatment with lasers. The effect of a particular laser on the skin is determined by optical qualities of skin components such as color or absorption characteristics, and by physical properties of the laser including wavelength, power, and duration of exposure (pulse width). Wavelength determines how far into the skin laser light will penetrate. The power of the laser and the duration of the pulse of laser light determine how much laser energy is imparted to the skin. These variables can be strategically selected and combined to provide a remarkable degree of precision, using the principle of selective photothermolysis. This principle underlies nearly all cosmetic lasers introduced in the past 15 years. New cosmetic lasers include nonsurgical machines, which remove a specific undesired skin component but do not alter overall skin structure, and surgical machines, which safely remove entire layers of skin without damaging the remaining skin but which require a period of healing. Nonsurgical lasers are used—without damaging the skin or changing its appearance in any way—to remove such unwanted skin features as tattoos, pigmented age spots, and birthmarks; vascular lesions including dilated blood vessels and port wine stains; and even excessive hair. The most common surgical cosmetic laser procedure is laser resurfacing, in which sun-damaged, aged superficial skin layers (including the entire epidermis and some of the dermis) are removed in a controlled fashion. Most of the improvement that follows is a result of the skin's remarkable ability to regenerate itself while healing, producing new tissue to replace what was removed by the laser.

Chromophores: the Actual "Targets" of Lasers

A chromophore (chromo = color, phore = carrier) is a chemical entity that absorbs a specific wavelength of the electromagnetic spectrum. In the skin, a chromophore is the target or skin component that is treated with a laser. Most skin chromophores have a distinct and intrinsic color. One of the major chromophores is melanin, the complex molecule largely responsible for the color of skin and hair. Most melanin is stored in tiny subcellular structures called melanosomes. Lasers used to remove excessive or unwanted skin color are optimized for energy absorption by melanin, the result of which is destruction of melanosomes or even of the cells that contain them—melanocytes.

Another major skin chromophore is hemoglobin in the red blood cells that are abundant within blood vessels and that are in close proximity to the walls of the vessels. Hemoglobin is the ideal chromophore to target if the goal is to damage or remove unwanted blood vessels, such as those that compose a vascular birthmark. The hemoglobin absorbs the laser energy, which is immediately converted to heat. In certain lasers such as the pulsed dye laser, a microscopic explosion literally blows apart the capillary. In other lasers such as the krypton laser, the heat damages the cells that line the blood vessel, resulting in coagulation of the blood in the vessel. Coagulation results in destruction and disappearance of the blood vessel.

Other common chromophores in the skin are the ink particles in a tattoo. Tattoo inks are foreign substances and generally differ in color and physical properties from natural skin components. Several lasers are designed to exploit the characteristics of tattoo ink. These ultra-short (5–100 nanoseconds; a nanosecond is one billionth of a

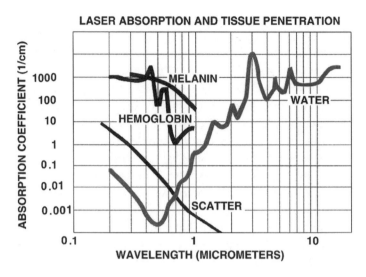

Fig. 4.1 Absorption spectra of the three major chromophores of human skin: melanin, hemoglobin, and water. Also depicted is scatter, a factor that strongly affects the depth to which light penetrates the skin. As wavelength of light increases, scattering decreases and depth of penetration increases.

second) pulsed lasers are so precise that they are capable of pulverizing ink particles while having no apparent effect on any natural skin components.

All colored objects absorb certain wavelengths of light and reflect others. For example, an object appears blue because it reflects blue light, absorbing all other colors. Each chromophore has a unique absorption spectrum, a pattern of light absorption at each of many wavelengths (fig. 4.1). The absorption spectrum is determined by illuminating a substance with light of different wavelengths and determining if that wavelength is absorbed or reflected. For pure substances there is frequently a complementariness to the colors, such that a red substance like hemoglobin will maximally absorb green light. Similarly, a red tattoo pigment will maximally absorb green light. A green chromophore, such as a green tattoo pigment, will maximally absorb red light. The ideal laser to affect a given target is the one maximally absorbed by that target.

The skin surface absorbs some light wavelengths and reflects others. The depth of penetration of absorbed light is largely determined by the wavelength of the light. In general, for visible light, the longer the wavelength, the deeper the penetration. Shorter wavelengths are much more likely to scatter, or change direction, essentially by reflecting off of tiny subcellular structures whose diameters are similar to the wavelength of visible light (fig. 4.1). Scattering is the main reason that shorter wavelengths are unable to penetrate deeply, and in the visible light spectrum (fig. 4.2), wavelengths shorter than about 500 nanometers (blue-green) are of little use in treating the skin because they barely penetrate the top layers of the epidermis.

A common wavelength used in nonsurgical lasers is 532 nanometers (nm). (A nanometer is one billionth of a meter; a meter is approximately 39 inches.) This is the wavelength produced by the frequency-doubled Nd:YAG laser and by certain diode lasers. This wavelength is green and is well absorbed by melanin. Because this relatively short wavelength does not penetrate very far into the skin, it is most effective at treating superficial pigmented lesions such as solar lentigenes (flat brown spots that occur in sun-exposed skin). These age spots are caused by excessive brown melanin pigment within the lowermost or basal layer of the epidermis (fig. 2.1).

Selective Photothermolysis: the Enabling Principle for Cosmetic Laser Surgery

The era of cosmetic laser treatment of the skin began in the 1980s with the work of Harvard University dermatologists Rox Anderson and John Parrish, who used laser energy to selectively damage dermal blood vessels. They considered the physical properties of small blood vessels, including their depth, diameter, laser energy absorption of their chromophore (hemoglobin), and thermal relaxation time, a measure of how quickly a structure cools down after being heated to a certain temperature. They theorized that a laser with a high energy level (fluence), a short pulse duration,

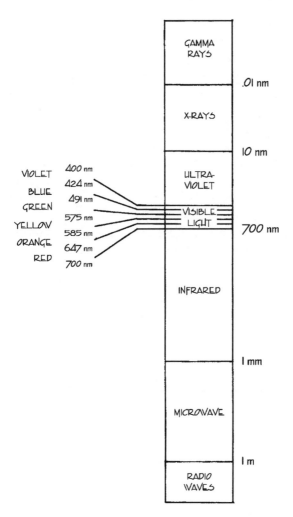

Fig. 4.2 The electromagnetic spectrum includes all wavelengths of electromagnetic radiation. Shorter wavelengths have higher energy. Visible light wavelengths range from about 400 nanometers (nm) to 700 nm. Ultraviolet "light" is invisible electromagnetic radiation with higher energy than violet light and wavelengths as short as 10 nm. Infrared radiation has lower energy than red light and wavelengths up to 1 millimeter (1 mm = 1 million nm). Radio waves have wavelengths greater than 1 meter (1 m = 1 billion nm).

and a wavelength that was highly absorbed by hemoglobin (relative to other skin chromophores) could be used. Pulse duration had to be shorter than thermal relaxation time so that heat would not build up excessively within the blood vessel and then be conducted to surrounding dermal tissue, causing a burn injury (with resultant scarring).

A good analogy of such limited thermal effect is a very brief contact of a finger with a hot pan on top of a kitchen stove. The pan could cause a severe burn if the skin were in contact with it for more than a split second. If the finger is immediately pulled away, insufficient heat energy is absorbed by the skin to cause a burn because the period of contact is so short.

Anderson and Parrish coined the term "selective photothermolysis" for their theory. A properly designed laser could cause *lysis* (damage or destruction) of a *selective* target through heat (*thermal* energy) generated by light (*photo*) from the laser. "Selective" is the key term: only the desired target should be affected. Only a laser could provide sufficient energy at a precise wavelength to enable selective photothermolysis.

A Brief History of Lasers Used to Treat Skin

In 1963 Leon Goldman, a dermatologist at the University of Cincinnati, used a laser for the first time on human skin. He used a ruby laser, which emits laser energy at 694 nm, in the red part of the visible light spectrum. This laser was a "normal mode" ruby laser that produced pulses of laser energy about one thousandth of a second in length. (This was very early in the laser era. The first laser ever built, in 1960, was also a ruby laser.) Dr. Goldman's laser produced only a low power beam. He and his colleagues were curious about the effect the laser might have on human skin. There was little effect on the skin at this low power level except for singeing of hairs and a mild burn effect.

The following year Dr. Goldman and his colleagues used a "Q-switched" ruby laser on a man with a dark blue tattoo. (The

Q-switch is a device in the laser cavity that includes a polarizing filter to block the passage of photons. The material in the laser cavity is kept in a highly excited state and then an electrical signal changes the polarity for an extremely short time, allowing the passage of light through the filter. The Q-switch is many thousands of times faster than any mechanical switch and produces a very high energy laser pulse of extremely short duration.) These researchers observed an immediate whitening of the treated tattoo and correctly surmised that this effect was something other than simple heating of the skin. There was only mild pain and no adverse effect on the skin. Although they did not know it at the time, their treatment of this tattoo was the first ever example of selective photothermolysis.

Surgical Lasers for Treating Skin

After Dr. Goldman's early efforts, the first truly useful lasers to treat skin disease were used to aid in surgery.

In the 1970s carbon dioxide (CO_2) lasers were developed for surgical use. (Most lasers are named after the chemical substance within the laser cavity responsible for producing the laser energy. In the case of the CO_2 laser, this substance is carbon dioxide, a gas. The specific wavelength of a given laser is determined by the energy levels of the electrons within the molecules of the chemical substance [see chapter 1].) The CO_2 laser has a wavelength of 10,600 nm, which is quite far into the infrared region of the electromagnetic spectrum, much longer than the wavelengths of visible light (400–700 nm, fig. 4.2). This wavelength is well absorbed by water molecules; thus, water acts as a chromophore for the CO_2 laser. Water is ubiquitous in human skin except for in the topmost cornified layer of the epidermis (stratum corneum). The viable layers of the epidermis, like nearly all living tissue, have a high water content and the dermis is composed primarily of water. Because there is so much water in skin, the effect of the CO_2 laser is not specific and treatment with this laser results in vaporization of all skin components;

the CO_2 laser is thus a surgical instrument because it alters the overall structure of the skin.

The first CO_2 lasers used for cutaneous surgery were continuous-wave devices; that is, the laser beam was on whenever the power switch was on. The duration of a pulse of energy from a continuous-wave laser is controlled by a mechanical switch, which has physical limitations as to how quickly it can be turned on and off. Because of the ubiquitous presence of water in tissues, a continuous-wave CO_2 laser always generates significant heat in the tissue being treated. This heating can be very beneficial for surgery because it coagulates the blood, which closes off the vessels. It is thus possible to perform "bloodless" surgery with the CO_2 laser. This destructive thermal effect is also desirable when treating skin cancers or tumors. Simple tissue destruction can also be achieved by non-laser technologies such as electrosurgery. Both the continuous-wave CO_2 laser and electrosurgery destroy tissue by producing very high temperatures (essentially burning the skin); the laser offers few advantages when simple tissue destruction is the goal.

In the 1980s, because of the bloodless nature of the continuous-wave CO_2 laser, surgeons thought that this instrument might be of value to cosmetic surgery. When the CO_2 laser beam is focused through lenses to a tiny area (0.1 to 0.2 mm), it is capable of slicing through tissue and can substitute for the traditional scalpel. The advantage of the CO_2 laser is most pronounced in cosmetic eyelid surgery (blepharoplasty). Eyelids have many small blood vessels and usually there is much bleeding and postoperative bruising when traditional scalpel methods are used. The focused continuous-wave CO_2 laser is able to cut through the tissue and seal blood vessels simultaneously. The result is little or no postoperative bruising and reduced swelling with laser blepharoplasty. The laser technique is also safer because postoperative bleeding in the eye area can be very dangerous and can even cause vision loss.

Scalpel surgery always results in copious bleeding, which usually requires the use of electrical cautery for control. Because the skin and other tissues have high content of water and salts, electrical currents can conduct beyond the immediate site to which they are applied, sometimes causing unforeseen damage. CO_2 laser energy, in contrast, is immediately absorbed and thus does not penetrate significantly beyond the surface on which it is used. This confined tissue effect is another advantage of the CO_2 laser over scalpel/electrosurgery techniques.

By the late 1980s, early attempts at resurfacing facial skin for the purpose of removing wrinkles were made using the CO_2 laser. Resurfacing facial skin with a continuous-wave CO_2 laser was a challenging proposition because the only way to achieve selective photothermolysis was to move the laser beam rapidly over the skin, avoiding a prolonged dwell time (remember the hot stove analogy discussed earlier in this chapter). Because of the risk of scarring, few surgeons were eager to attempt facial resurfacing with the continuous-wave CO_2 laser.

In the early 1990s, the UltraPulse CO_2 laser was introduced. The UltraPulse technology enabled very high-energy laser output delivered during a very brief (one millisecond: one thousandth of a second) pulse. For the first time, selective photothermolysis was possible with a CO_2 laser. I first heard of this new technology in June 1992 at the inaugural meeting of the International Society of Cosmetic Laser Surgeons (ISCLS). Dr. Richard Fitzpatrick, a dermatologist from San Diego, CA, reported using the UltraPulse laser to remove pre-cancerous skin lesions (solar keratoses). To his surprise, after healing, these patients also demonstrated significant improvement in facial wrinkles. Dr. Fitzpatrick coined the term "laser resurfacing" to describe this new technique. Laser resurfacing was the procedure most responsible for the rapid growth of cosmetic laser surgery during the 1990s.

In the mid-1990s a new, even more precise laser was introduced for skin resurfacing: the erbium:YAG laser. This laser is similar to the CO_2 laser in that its chromophore in the skin is water, and its wavelength is in the infrared region of the electromagnetic spectrum. The special properties of the erbium:YAG laser are due to its wavelength, 2940 nm, which almost exactly matches the highest peak of the absorption spectrum for the water molecule (fig. 4.1). At 2940 nm water absorbs over ten times as much energy as it does at the wavelength of the CO_2 laser, 10,600 nm. This means that nearly all of the laser energy is consumed by heating water, thus vaporizing tissue, and very little energy is left to scatter into the skin and produce nonspecific heating. The residual thermal effect of the erbium:YAG laser is negligble because it produces nearly pure tissue ablation (removal).

The lack of nonspecific heating from the erbium:YAG laser offers several advantages for laser resurfacing. These include less pain, faster healing (30–50% faster than with CO_2 laser resurfacing) and less redness of the skin after healing. The major disadvantage of the erbium:YAG laser is that, unlike the CO_2 laser, it does not seal blood vessels in the dermis. Thus, bleeding during resurfacing can be a problem for the surgeon unless appropriate topically applied medications are used to cause blood vessel constriction (see chapter 6). Remarkably, the erbium:YAG laser is "as good as it gets" when it comes to resurfacing, because its wavelength nearly perfectly matches the highest level of absorption for water. Because of its wavelength the erbium:YAG laser will probably stand as the technological standard for laser resurfacing for many years.

Nonsurgical Lasers for Treating Skin

One of the first clinical applications of selective photothermolysis was the pulsed dye laser. The first model was developed at the Candela Corporation of Massachusetts in 1983. This laser was engineered to selectively treat abnormal blood vessels in the skin. The primary objective of the first pulsed dye laser was to treat port wine stains, a type of birthmark composed of a patch of skin with a greatly increased density of capillaries (tiny blood vessels), enough to impart a permanent, intense red color. (Port wine stains arise in childhood and can be emotionally devastating if present in cosmetically sensitive areas such as the face or distal [exposed] extremities. In these lesions, the skin generally has a normal texture and in fact is normal except for the dense concentration of capillaries.) These excessive capillaries serve no physiologic function and can be removed completely from the skin without causing any harm.

Prior to the development of the pulsed dye laser, the argon laser was the best option for treating blood vessels. Introduced in the 1970s, the argon laser produces blue-green light with a wavelength of 514 nm. This color is well absorbed by the hemoglobin molecule in red blood cells and is near a peak in the absorption spectrum of hemoglobin (fig. 4.1), and thus has a selective effect on vascular tissue. This laser was used primarily by ophthalmologists to destroy abnormal blood vessels in the retina that occur in diseases such as diabetes and can lead to blindness if untreated. The argon laser was used with some success to treat cutaneous blood vessels. Most responsive were large facial vessels (telangiectases), which are common in people with the acne-like skin disease rosacea and can also occur in people who have had excessive chronic sun exposure. The physical and optical properties of port wine stains are different from those of telangiectases such that treating them with the argon laser was quite difficult. The laser characteristics effective in destroying the capillaries would also very likely damage the skin enough to cause a burn and a scar. The problems with the argon laser included a wavelength that was too short to enable adequate depth of penetration into the skin (thus not reaching the deeper capillaries of a port wine stain) and a pulse duration that was too long to result in selective photothermolysis.

The engineers at Candela Corporation tried to improve on the argon laser with a new laser design that enabled a very short pulse (less than half a millisecond). This laser was powered by a flash lamp: a bright electric lamp that flashed on for a brief time. The laser cavity contained a dye dissolved in alcohol. The dye was an organic compound and could be altered in such a way that the laser wavelength could be changed. The laser was thus tunable and could generate different wavelengths. It was called a "flash lamp-pumped tunable dye laser" or a "pulsed dye laser."

Consulting with dermatologists, these engineers tried different laser wavelengths to treat port wine stains. They found significant differences in treatment response with changes in wavelength as little as a few nanometers. Ultimately, the most effective wavelength for the majority of port wine stains was 585 nm. This wavelength is close to the absorption peak of hemoglobin (fig. 4.1) but is long enough to penetrate into the dermis, the skin level in which the blood vessels are located. This deeper penetration, combined with short pulse duration, gave the pulsed dye laser significant advantages in both efficacy and safety compared to the older argon laser.

Because telangiectases are relatively superficial, they can be effectively treated with shorter laser wavelengths than those required for port wine stains. Even continuous lasers such as the argon, the krypton, and newer green light (532 nm) diode lasers can be used with mechanically switched pulses (0.05 to 0.10 seconds) to safely remove these vessels. These continuous lasers require careful use because too long a pulse duration and/or too high a power level could damage the skin. When used properly, these lasers produce a practical selective photothermolysis because the unwanted vessels can be removed without damaging other skin components. Two additional lasers that are somewhat less common than the argon and krypton laser and that produce similar clinical results are the copper vapor and copper bromide lasers.

Q-Switched Lasers

In the early 1980s, Q-switched lasers were first successfully used for cosmetic applications in medicine. A Q-switch is a type of chemical switch that is much faster than any mechanical switch. With Q-switching, laser pulses as brief as 5 nanoseconds are possible. The first published report on the use of the Q-switched ruby laser (694 nm) to treat a series of patients with tattoos appeared in 1983. This laser was found to work well on black and green tattoo inks. Subsequently, other visible and near-infrared wavelength Q-switched lasers (Nd:YAG, alexandrite) were developed. These lasers produce wavelengths that are absorbed by other chromophores; this feature as well as the very high-energy and ultrashort pulses of the Q-switched lasers enable effective photothermolysis of a variety of tattoo inks.

The exact process of clearance of tattoo ink appears to involve shattering of the ink particles. The pulverized fragments are ingested by macrophages (a type of white blood cell), and the tattoo ink actually disappears from the skin. The incidence of scarring or skin damage is extremely low with Q-switched laser treatment for tattoos; this is thus a nonsurgical treatment. In contrast, surgical treatments for tattoos invariably result in significant scarring.

Q-switched lasers are also useful for treating benign pigmented lesions such as lentigenes. Because melanin absorbs a broad range of wavelengths, several Q-switched lasers are effective at removing excessive melanin. In different pigmented lesions, the excess melanin is present at different levels in the skin. In lentigenes, the melanin is within the epidermis; it is effectively treated with short wavelength Q-switched lasers such as the frequency doubled Nd:YAG (532 nm) and ruby (694 nm) lasers. Certain pigmented birthmarks have excess melanin deeper in the dermis. The Q-switched Nd:YAG laser (1064 nm) is effective at treating these deeper lesions because its long wavelength light penetrates farther into the dermis.

Hair Removal Lasers

In the late 1990s, new lasers were developed for the purpose of removing unwanted hair. All of these lasers target the chromophore melanin, which in dark hair is present at greater concentrations in the hair follicle than in the surrounding skin. White or gray hair follicles cannot be treated as effectively because they lack melanin. Most of the lasers used for hair removal are similar to the Q-switched lasers (ruby, alexandrite, Nd:YAG) but are run in normal mode with pulses of laser energy much longer than those generated by a Q-switch. The longer pulses are needed to impart sufficient energy to the hair follicle to cause its destruction. Many of these laser systems require simultaneous use of a skin coolant to protect the epidermis, with its lower melanin content, from excessive heating. Ironically, cutaneous lasers seem to have come full circle since the original work of Dr. Leon Goldman, who used a normal mode ruby laser for the first ever laser treatment of human skin.

The history of lasers used to improve the skin's appearance is one of continuous refinement in technology in order to meet the demanding requirements of cosmetic surgery: the destruction or removal of unwanted skin elements without harming the skin. Improvement in laser design is made possible through increased understanding of the skin's physical properties and through ingenious engineering to take advantage of these properties. In the next two chapters we will discuss the topic of greatest interest to any prospective patient: what is it like to be treated with a laser?

5. What Is It Like to Be Treated with a Nonsurgical Laser?

A patient about to undergo laser treatment might wonder what the experience will be like. Will it hurt? Is it dangerous? Will there be any anesthesia injections? How long does it take to heal?

As might be expected, there is a significant difference between nonsurgical and surgical laser treatments. For the most part, nonsurgical laser treatments have a more limited effect on the skin because the laser energy is absorbed by a targeted skin component. Only the unwanted skin components, such as blood vessels, pigmented cells or hair follicles, are damaged. With nonsurgical laser treatments pain is mild; usually no anesthesia is required. In contrast, surgical laser treatments are nonspecific and affect all skin components equally. In laser resurfacing, entire layers of skin are removed and significant healing must take place because new skin must grow to replace the removed skin. Incisional laser surgery requires stitches to close the wound.

Removing Vascular Skin Lesions

In younger patients, port wine stains are usually composed of superficial capillaries, whereas in adults they may also include larger, darker blood vessels. Lesions that are composed primarily of capillaries respond best to pulsed dye laser treatment; those with larger vessels may also require treatment with a continuous-wave laser, such as the krypton, argon, or normal mode Nd:YAG lasers.

Pulsed dye laser therapy is moderately painful. The painful sensation is felt briefly during each laser pulse. In older children or adults, anesthesia is usually not required. Younger children or infants generally will not tolerate this level of pain and thus cannot cooperate during treatment. Therefore, pulsed dye laser treatment may require sedation or even general anesthesia in this age group.

Pulsed dye laser treatment of vascular lesions generally results in purpura, an immediate bruise-like discoloration that occurs due to a shock wave effect. (Newer pulsed dye lasers with slightly longer pulse durations are less likely to cause purpura.) The high-energy, brief laser pulse is highly absorbed by hemoglobin within red blood cells and is converted to heat. This heat absorption causes rapid expansion and results in microscopic explosions within the capillaries, physically disrupting the walls of the small blood vessels so that red blood cell contents (primarily hemoglobin) leak out of the vessels into the surrounding dermis. The bruise-like purpura will fade as macrophages remove this debris, but may require up to two weeks to completely disappear. In addition to purpura, the microscopic injury to blood vessels may cause inflammation that results in mild swelling of the treated skin.

Unlike port wine stains, hemangiomas are raised, fleshy growths composed mostly of larger, dilated blood vessels. Some port wine stains are actually mixed lesions that include small hemangiomas within the larger flat port wine stain. Hemangiomas generally show only a partial response to treatment with the pulsed dye laser; the blood vessels within a hemangioma are too large to be destroyed by the shock wave effect of the pulsed dye laser. All of the energy in the laser pulse is absorbed by hemoglobin within the red blood cells adjacent to the proximal vessel wall. Although there may be disruption to part of the vessel wall, the vessel wall will heal and the vessel will survive.

A method more effective in destroying the larger vessels of a hemangioma is a continuous-wave laser such as the argon or krypton laser. These lasers produce energy at wavelengths that are well absorbed by hemoglobin and can be operated in a truly continuous mode or mechanically switched to provide pulses as short as five-hundredths of a second. These longer pulses generate sufficient heat within the vessels to cause coagulation of the blood. A coagulated vessel dies and will disappear as macrophages remove the resultant debris.

Treatment of small (one-eighth inch or less) hemangiomas with krypton or argon lasers is relatively painless and requires no anesthesia. Very small lesions will shrink and disappear immediately, healing with no visible scar. Larger lesions may turn gray and heal by forming a scab. A scab forms because the epidermis overlying the hemangioma is destroyed and the blood within the hemangioma, now coagulated, is on the surface. (A scab is dried, coagulated blood on the surface of the skin.)

Larger hemangiomas are more difficult and painful to treat. These lesions may require an injected anesthetic before treatment. The laser energy may need to be administered through repeated pulses or even continuous, non-pulsed treatment. Large lesions, because of their size, absorb a large amount of laser energy and are heated to a relatively high temperature. If enough heat is conducted to adjacent skin, there will be a localized burn, possibly resulting in a wound that heals with a visible scar. Because continuous-wave lasers such as krypton and argon produce coagulation within targeted blood vessels, there is no purpura. In the days following treatment, there may be superficial crusting or scabbing to which a topical antibiotic such as bacitracin or Polysporin should be applied once or twice a day.

A telangiectasia is a visibly dilated, linear blood vessel. Telangiectases, which may be associated with a diffuse redness or blush due to accompanying microscopic capillaries, occur primarily on the face and may be associated with a skin disease such as rosacea. Rosacea is an acne-like condition that occurs in adults. People with rosacea experience frequent flushing (blushing) of facial skin. During flushing, facial blood vessels dilate, producing visible redness. Many vessels eventually become permanently dilated (telangiectases). Telangiectases also frequently occur as a consequence of excessive sun exposure.

Because they are small, facial telangiectases may respond to treatment with the pulsed dye laser. This laser is more likely to work on small-diameter vessels and capillaries and usually produces purpura, which may persist as long as two weeks after treatment. Krypton, argon, and 532 nm diode lasers are useful for treating telangiectases and have the advantage of not producing purpura. For this reason, most patients prefer these over the pulsed dye laser. None of these lasers require anesthesia in the great majority of patients. The final result of a treatment may not be apparent for several weeks.

After treatment with the krypton or argon laser the blood within many of the telangiectases will undergo coagulation, so blood flow within the vessels stops. Once the blood within a vessel coagulates, the body disposes of the vessel's remains and the vessel is obliterated.

Removing Brown Pigmented Lesions

Several types of lasers are effective for treating lentigenes because melanin absorbs light of many wavelengths. Anesthesia is generally not required. The lesions may turn a gray or whitish color immediately upon treatment. There may be an additional purple discoloration (purpura) upon treatment with the Q-switched Nd:YAG laser. This purpura is caused by a shock wave effect on nearby blood vessels similar to that produced by the pulsed dye laser. Other lasers used for treating lentigenes are Q-switched ruby and alexandrite lasers, and continuous-wave krypton and diode lasers.

Other flat pigmented lesions, including freckles and cafe-au-lait spots, are treated the same way as lentigenes. All are likely to fade completely with one or two treatments. Darker lesions tend to respond better than lighter ones because they absorb more laser energy. Very light pigmented lesions absorb less laser energy, possibly not enough to cause significant damage to the pigment cells. For unknown reasons, cafe-au-lait spots are quite likely to recur within a few months and may require repeated treatments.

Melanocytic nevi (moles) are commonly considered for cosmetic removal. Because melanocytic nevus cells have the potential to become malignant, they must be dealt with cautiously. For many years the standard approach to removing nevi has been surgical excision. One advantage of surgical removal is that the tissue can be processed and examined microscopically by a pathologist. Pathologic analysis confirms whether the cells are benign or malignant. Indeed, a biopsy should be obtained from any mole that is suggestive of being abnormal, to enable pathologic assessment. Moles that appear normal but that are cosmetically objectionable to the patient may be considered for laser removal. A skilled dermatologist should make the judgment as to whether it is safe to remove a nevus with a laser. In many cases, laser treatments of nevi provide superior cosmetic results compared to conventional surgical excision.

Small nevi judged to be benign can be removed by laser vaporization (CO_2 or erbium:YAG laser). I often remove small nevi that are within a facial area that I am resurfacing with one of these lasers. I have also found the krypton laser to be effective for removing small pigmented nevi. In these lesions the pigment preferentially absorbs the green light output of the krypton laser, concentrating the thermal damage in the nevus cells. All of these lasers may be somewhat painful on treatment and may require an injected local anesthetic. The treated lesion will usually heal with a scab over a period of one or two weeks.

Treating larger nevi (greater than one-eighth inch in diameter) with a destructive laser is more risky because there is a greater chance of scarring. Depending on the body area, surgical excision, which always creates a scar, may be cosmetically superior to laser removal. One type of large nevus best treated with a laser is the nevus of Ota (see chapter 2). This is a pigmented lesion composed of nevus cells that lie deep in the dermis. These lesions are usually several inches in diameter. The color varies in intensity (based on the amount of pigment) and hue (based on the depth of pigment in the dermis). Q-switched lasers have been found to be most effective for treating nevi of Ota. Deeper pigment responds better to the Q-switched Nd:YAG laser, whereas more superficial pigment may require the Q-switched ruby laser. These nonsurgical treatments are generally done without anesthesia. Multiple treatments are required.

Laser Treatment of Tattoos

Black is the most responsive tattoo ink and responds equally well to all three Q-switched lasers. Black ink particles absorb all visible wavelengths. Red ink requires treatment with the frequency-doubled (532 nm) Q-switched Nd:YAG laser. Green responds to Q-switched ruby (694 nm) and alexandrite (755 nm) lasers and can also be treated with the Q-switched Nd:YAG laser using a special handpiece that alters the wavelength of the laser energy to 650 nm. Dark blue ink may respond as black ink does. Yellow tattoo ink is relatively resistant to all laser wavelengths but is generally inconspicuous if it remains after the other tattoo colors have cleared.

The great advantage of Q-switched lasers is that they are very safe; the risk of adverse events such as scarring is extremely low. Many tattoos can be completely eradicated with no visible effect on the skin. The disadvantage is that most tattoos require multiple treatments. In contrast, a surgical treatment (such as the CO_2 laser) may provide drastic reduction in the tattoo after only one treatment but will always cause a significant scar, which usually looks worse than the tattoo.

Amateur-applied tattoos usually contain less ink and will therefore clear with fewer treatments, frequently four or fewer. Professional tattoos require six or more treatments and, if multicolored, may need many more. There will be a differential clearance of ink based on color. Black ink may be completely cleared while more resistant inks remain quite prominent. In recent years novel colors have been appearing in tattoos. These newer inks are typically brighter than traditional tattoo ink and occur in a wider array of colors. Such novel colors are less likely than conventional colors to respond to Q-switched laser treatments. One should have low expectations for laser treatment of bright, multicolored tattoos; however, such tattoos may clear if given a greater number of treatments. Dr. Rox Anderson, the co-discoverer of selective photothermolysis (the principle that enables nonsurgical laser removal of tattoos), has proposed restriction of tattoo inks to those that are known to be responsive to Q-switched laser treatment. (The U.S. Food and Drug

Administration regulates tattoo inks as cosmetics and the pigments used in them as color additives. The actual use of tattoo inks is not regulated at the federal level but rather in local jurisdictions.)

Two additional factors seem to affect the responsiveness of tattoos to Q-switched laser treatment: the age of the tattoo (time elapsed since the tattoo was obtained) and the body location of the tattoo. In general, older tattoos seem somewhat more responsive than newer tattoos. The reason for this difference may be that the body's efforts to clear the tattoo ink have actually begun to have an effect. (Remember that the laser breaks up tattoo ink particles and that the body's macrophage cells remove the particle fragments; see chapter 4.) As for body location, more distal locations on an extremity (such as the hand or foot) appear to respond less rapidly than proximal extremities (upper arm, thigh) or trunk locations. Also, lower body locations are less responsive than upper body locations (one can surmise that the worst body location would be the foot). The effect of body location on a tattoo's response to treatment may be related to blood circulation, which is better in the more responsive locations.

Q-switched laser treatment of tattoos is moderately painful but usually does not require anesthesia. These extremely short-pulsed lasers produce a sensation similar to that of a rubber band snapping against the skin. The sensation is sharp but very brief, and is painful mainly during the actual treatment. Topical anesthetic creams such as EMLA or Betacaine may be partially helpful but are limited in effect because they numb only the more superficial layers of skin. Unfortunately, it is the deeper layers (in the dermis) where the tattoo ink particles are located. Subsequent laser treatments are progressively less painful because there is less and less ink in the tattoo. In fact, where there is no tattoo ink in the skin, these lasers are virtually painless. This is because tattooed skin contains much more chromophore than does normal skin.

Initial treatment of a dark tattoo may produce an exuberant reaction in which the absorbed laser energy produces a small shock wave effect. This is commonly felt as a vibration in the skin and may be enough to actually disrupt the epidermis above the tattoo, producing pinpoint bleeding. This effect should not be confused with that of a surgical treatment, however, because this type of minor skin disruption will heal very quickly. The physician may suggest that the patient apply topical antibiotic ointment, such as bacitracin, to any minor scabs that may appear in the first few days following treatment.

Laser Hair Removal

Hair removal lasers all target melanin. Unwanted hairs tend to be relatively large and dark. There is a much higher concentration of melanin in the hair follicle than in the surrounding skin; this difference provides selectivity so that the laser's effect is much greater on the hair follicle than elsewhere. Human hair varies widely in diameter and color as well as in growth characteristics; the response to laser hair removal treatment is affected by all of these physical features.

Because of the broad range of wavelengths that affect melanin (see chapter 4), several different lasers are effective for hair removal: ruby (694 nm), alexandrite (755 nm), diode (810 nm), and Nd:YAG (1064 nm) lasers. These lasers have variable power settings, spot sizes and pulse durations, all of which can affect the efficacy of treatment. The hair follicle is a relatively large structure, and significant amounts of energy are required to damage it; a relatively long laser pulse is required to deliver the needed energy. To avoid excessive heating of the epidermis, a cooling agent is generally used. Examples of cooling techniques include application of an ice-cold gel, a block of frozen blue ice, or a refrigerant spray. Laser treatment follows this cooling step. These coolants chill the epidermis more than the dermis, so that the laser treatment primarily affects the dermis, the location of the hair follicle.

Most modern hair removal lasers employ a large spot size (half an inch or more in diameter); this entire circular area is treated with one laser pulse. Ideally the tissue damage is confined to the hair follicles and the rest of the skin is unharmed. Because the laser pulses may be produced at the rate of one or more per second, an entire upper lip area may be treated in less than 30 seconds. The laser affects all growing hair follicles in the treated area. Pain is relatively mild and is actually lessened by chilling of the skin (cold has an anesthetic effect). Generally no anesthetics are required. The relative speed of laser hair removal enables treatment of large body areas such as legs, arms and trunk. These areas are often several hundred times greater than that of the upper lip and may require 30 to 60 minutes to treat. Such long treatments consequently involve more pain.

Electrolysis is the only other truly destructive method of hair removal and should be compared to laser hair removal. Both methods can result in permanent effects. In electrolysis, a tiny electrode is placed down each individual hair follicle. There is significant pain with each electrical impulse. These treatments are slow and tedious; an upper lip may require an hour or more for complete treatment. (In practice, few people can tolerate more than 30 minutes of treatment in a single session.) The success of electrolysis is highly dependent on the skill of the technician and varies widely. In addition, there is a risk of scarring with over-treatment. In contrast, laser hair removal is extremely fast and relatively painless. Laser treatments are largely standardized and success is somewhat independent of the skills of the operator. In patients with lighter skin, over-treatment that results in scarring is uncommon. Caution must be exercised when treating patients with darker skin types. This is because with greater amounts of melanin in the epidermis there is a higher risk of unwanted heating of the epidermis. Extensive epidermal heating may result in temporary or permanent changes in pigmentation (either hyper- or hypo-pigmentation) or even a scar (a permanent change in texture).

As we have seen, nonsurgical laser treatments precisely remove unwanted skin elements by targeting specific skin chromophores. Ideally these treatments affect only the unwanted elements, cause no damage to the rest of the skin and therefore require little if any visible healing, and result in no scarring or changes in skin texture. In contrast, surgical laser treatments target a universal chromophore (water) that is present throughout the skin, and are intended to vaporize (remove) entire layers of skin or to excise (cut through) skin and other soft tissues. As I shall discuss in the next chapter, the special properties of lasers can be used to great advantage by cosmetic surgeons.

6. What Is It Like to Be Treated with a Surgical Laser?

Surgical treatment alters the structure of the skin, usually through removal of tissue, and thus requires a period of healing. Most surgical laser treatments are similar to conventional non-laser surgeries except that, instead of a mechanical abrading device or scalpel, a laser is used to remove or cut through tissue. Surgical lasers have special advantages in cosmetic surgery, such as sealing blood vessels and causing skin contraction, that are lacking in conventional surgical treatments. As with any cosmetic surgery, the quality of the result is highly dependent on the skill of the surgeon.

Laser Resurfacing

Resurfacing of facial skin is the most common surgical laser treatment. These treatments are effective because they remove whole layers of sun-damaged skin; with healing, completely new skin actually replaces what was removed. Unwanted textural features such as wrinkles are smoothed out and, because the epidermis is entirely removed with resurfacing, age spots and splotchy pigmentation are also removed.

There are two types of resurfacing lasers in common use: erbium:YAG and CO_2. The energy output of each of these lasers is absorbed by water. Because water is everywhere in the skin, these lasers do not have an effect on a specific cell type or skin component but rather affect all skin components equally. These lasers are designed to treat a broad area of skin with each pulse or pass, each of which removes a uniform depth of tissue. Many models of resurfacing lasers use robotic scanners that facilitate uniform and rapid treatment of relatively large surface areas. Although the general principles of resurfacing with erbium:YAG and CO_2 lasers are similar, there are significant differences between them. Each laser has advantages and disadvantages.

The erbium:YAG laser has an extremely high affinity for water; almost all of this laser's energy is absorbed by water, resulting in immediate and complete vaporization of thin layers of skin. The fraction of laser energy not absorbed by water produces a small amount of residual heat in adjacent (lower) layers of skin. In contrast, the CO_2 laser has a lower affinity for water: in addition to vaporizing skin cells, this laser leaves a zone of heated skin below the vaporized skin layers. This residual heat is generally below the threshold to cause damage (that is, the skin does not suffer a burn injury), but it is enough to significantly affect the skin during and after healing. This residual heating effect accounts for all of the differences between CO_2 and erbium:YAG laser treatments. These differences include the amount of pain experienced during treatment, the possibility of bleeding during or after treatment, how much the skin contracts with treatment (immediate and delayed), how long it takes to heal, how much redness occurs after treatment, and the risk of alterations of skin pigmentation.

Laser Resurfacing with the Erbium:YAG Laser

Because erbium:YAG laser energy is almost completely consumed by vaporization of skin cells, resurfacing with this laser is substantially less painful than with the CO_2 laser. Although erbium:YAG resurfacing is not painless, the majority of facial areas can be treated using only topically applied anesthetic. Several effective anesthetic creams are available. Most provide better anesthesia if applied for longer periods prior to erbium:YAG laser resurfacing. One topical anesthetic, EMLA cream, usually requires two or more hours of application for maximal effectiveness. EMLA also works better if the cream is covered with a plastic film. If EMLA is used, patients are instructed to apply the cream before arriving at the physician's office. Other topical anesthetics, such as ElaMax and Betacaine, work more rapidly.

I studied Betacaine as an anesthetic for erbium:YAG laser resurfacing over a period of 18 months and reported the results at the 1999 meeting of the American Society for Lasers in Medicine and Surgery. Betacaine was used in 70 consecutive patients who underwent erbium:YAG laser resurfacing of facial areas during this period. Resurfacing was done for the purpose of smoothing wrinkles as well as scars from acne and chickenpox. Of 178 facial areas treated, 160 were adequately anesthetized with only the topical Betacaine. Facial areas that failed topical anesthesia were numbed using injected anesthetics at the patient's request. In this study, the overall success rate of topical anesthesia for erbium:YAG laser resurfacing was 95%. Fig. 6.1 shows before and after photographs of one of the patients treated in this study. Note that with proper technique even deep wrinkles can be removed completely with the erbium:YAG laser.

Most patients are pleased to hear that no injections are required for erbium:YAG laser resurfacing. For many patients this treatment is not painless, however, and they might prefer an anesthesia injection. The experience of pain is subjective and varies with an individual's pain threshold.

Another difference between erbium:YAG and CO_2 laser resurfacing is that there may be minor bleeding with the erbium:YAG treatment. The excess residual heat produced by the CO_2 laser will cause immediate coagulation of the small blood vessels in the skin, so there is generally no bleeding during CO_2 laser resurfacing. In contrast, the lack of residual heat in the treated skin during erbium: YAG resurfacing may result in mild bleeding. This bleeding is easily controlled by immediate application (by the surgeon) of a solution of aluminum chloride. In the hours following resurfacing there may be intermittent minor bleeding.

Contraction of the skin during erbium:YAG laser resurfacing is minimal compared to CO_2 laser resurfacing. Collagen, the major protein constituent of the dermis (see chapter 2), immediately shrinks if heated above a threshold temperature. The minimal residual heating

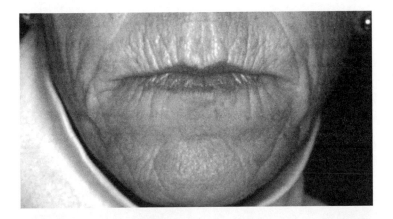

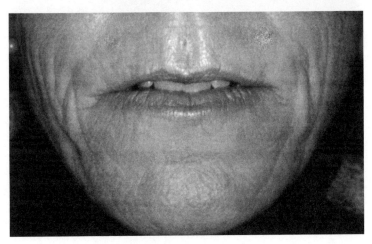

Fig. 6.1 This patient had deep wrinkles in the area around the mouth. She is shown before and after resurfacing with the erbium laser.

of treated skin by the erbium:YAG laser is below the threshold of collagen contraction. In contrast, the CO_2 laser produces considerable collagen shrinkage.

The erbium:YAG laser is particularly useful in resurfacing facial skin that is scarred from acne or chicken pox (fig. 6.2). The lack of contraction (and distortion) of the skin during erbium:YAG laser

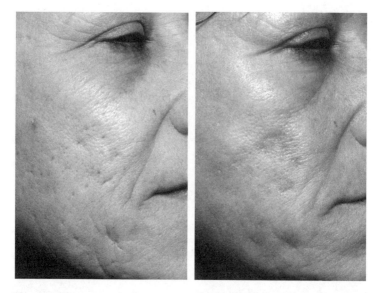

Fig. 6.2 This patient had acne scars of Types I and II. Some of the Type II acne scars on this patient were removed by punch excision. Then, using only topically applied anesthesia, erbium laser resurfacing was done on the acne scars and on the wrinkles around the eye. She is shown before and after treatment.

resurfacing enables the surgeon to precisely sculpt the scar tissue. The relative high points of elevated scar tissue are flattened to more closely match the low points. The ability to use only topical anesthetics during erbium:YAG laser resurfacing is also advantageous, because injected anesthetic solutions distort the skin's topology, artificially smoothing out scars and obscuring them from the surgeon's view. Because only a small amount of skin is removed with each pass of the erbium:YAG laser beam over the treated area, multiple passes (frequently five, ten, or more) with this laser are generally administered during a resurfacing session. After each of these laser passes, additional anesthetic solution is applied directly to the skin, thus increasing the anesthetic effect.

The end point of properly performed erbium:YAG laser resurfacing is when wrinkles or scars are largely or completely erased and the skin is smooth. When resurfacing is finished, a special flexible and very thin dressing (Flexzan) is applied directly to the treated area. This dressing is generally left in place during the next several days as the skin heals. Flexzan is opaque and has the advantage of obscuring the healing skin. It is obvious that the patient has a dressing on, however. Patients who do not want co-workers to know about their surgery will not return to work until after they have healed.

The benchmark of healing is reappearance of the epidermis (re-epithelialization). This healing process is relatively fast after erbium:YAG laser resurfacing and is generally complete within five to seven days. The continuous coverage provided by the occlusive dressing provides an optimal environment for rapid healing and also diminishes any painful sensation. The dressing protects healing skin from the environment. Water is repelled by the surface of the dressing, enabling showers or washing of the face. Patients who have an increased number of blood vessels in the treated skin area may experience some mild bleeding beneath the dressing in the hours following surgery.

When the dressing is removed, there may be small amounts of crust (dried blood or serum) on the surface. This material generally comes off in the next day or two when the face is washed. The newly healed skin is vulnerable to abrasion for several days and should be washed with a mild cleanser using only the hands (no washcloth). Most patients are able to return to work within seven to ten days of erbium:YAG laser resurfacing.

Red or pink color is a universal feature of healing skin and is to be expected after erbium:YAG (and CO_2) laser resurfacing. This color (termed erythema) is due to dilated capillaries. Capillaries dilate during wound healing, and the degree and duration of erythema after laser resurfacing is significantly less with the erbium:YAG than with the CO_2 laser. Like all other differences between these lasers, this is because of the relatively minimal heating of the skin from the erbium:YAG laser. For most people, this color is more pink than red and fades rapidly over the next few weeks; frequently the color is normal within one month. Facial areas with deeper wrinkles, which require more intensive treatment, will have greater and longer-lasting erythema. Most women prefer wearing makeup to cover the pink color and may do so within one week of the resurfacing procedure. Makeup effective for this purpose is widely available.

Sun protection is advisable after any skin resurfacing procedure. The skin's pigment system tends to overreact to the sun's ultraviolet light and to produce excessive amounts of melanin—an exaggerated tanning response (see chapter 2). This overproduction of melanin pigment, which can occur anytime the skin is inflamed (including in the first few weeks after resurfacing), is termed "post-inflammatory hyperpigmentation." The best approach to this problem is prevention through sun avoidance and the use of sunscreens (broad spectrum, SPF 30 or greater). If hyperpigmentation does occur, treatment with bleaching creams may be required. This condition usually responds well to such treatment.

One of the greatest safety features of the erbium:YAG laser is its relatively low risk of causing long-term pigmentary alterations—almost always hypopigmentation, or lightening of the treated skin. Hypopigmentation is uncommon after erbium:YAG laser resurfacing but is one of the most worrisome side effects of CO_2 laser resurfacing. Pigmentary lightening occurs more often in people with darker skin tones and, like all other differences between the erbium:YAG and CO_2 lasers, is attributable to the greater heating of the skin from the CO_2 laser. In certain people, melanocytes are sensitive to this heating and may fail to repopulate the epidermis after re-epithelialization or, if present, may underproduce melanin. In my opinion, the risk of hypopigmentation is the most important reason that partial face resurfacing should be done with the erbium:YAG rather than the CO_2 laser. Conversely, if the CO_2 laser is to be used, the entire face should be resurfaced. I have never seen objectionable hypopigmentation after CO_2 laser resurfacing of the entire face.

Laser Resurfacing with the CO_2 Laser

I reserve the CO_2 laser for full-face resurfacing. The goal of full-face resurfacing is to obtain maximum improvement of photo-aged skin. Many patients who consider full-face laser resurfacing are also considering a facelift. These patients are interested in significant improvement and realize that real changes are possible with a serious investment in cosmetic surgery. In patients whose skin has suffered extensive sun damage, full-face laser resurfacing may provide more impressive rejuvenation than that of a facelift.

In a facelift (rhytidectomy), the superficial fascia layer of the cheeks (immediately beneath the skin and fat layers) is pulled upward and outward toward the ear (see chapter 3). This fascia layer is tightened with stitches to counteract the gravitational sagging of the neck and lower facial area. After the superficial fascia is tightened, excess skin is cut out and the skin is stitched together in front of and behind the ear. Because the skin of the neck and lower cheeks is attached to the superficial fascia, the skin in these areas will appear tightened and less wrinkled after a facelift.

Many patients are concerned about the deep furrow that runs from the nose to the corner of the mouth (nasolabial fold) and seek a facelift partly to lessen this furrow. Unfortunately, a facelift has little effect on this furrow or several other areas of the face including the forehead, frown lines, crow's feet wrinkles of the temples, and wrinkles in the upper lip and chin areas. Wrinkles and aged skin in these areas do not improve from a facelift. Because a facelift is not a treatment for the skin, uneven skin pigmentation (blotches) are not affected anywhere on the face.

The more photodamage a patient has, the more improvement they can expect from full-face CO_2 laser resurfacing. With one procedure, the superficial skin layers are entirely renewed and the skin significantly tightens. This tightening is most evident in the cheeks (the facial area with the largest surface area). Contraction of cheek skin results in lessening of the nasolabial fold, frequently to a greater extent than does the fascia tightening of a facelift procedure.

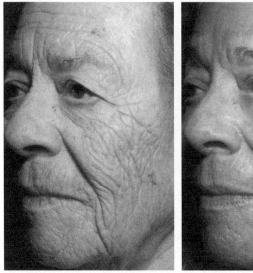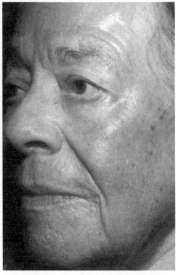

Fig. 6.3 This 87-year-old patient with severe photo-aging is shown before and two months after full face laser resurfacing with the CO_2 and erbium lasers. Notice the tightening of the skin resulting in elevation of the eyebrow and improvement in the deep folds around the mouth. Only local anesthesia was used.

Anatomical studies have demonstrated that tightening of the cheek skin diminishes the depth of this fold more than does tightening of the deeper fascia layer. With expert surgical technique, full-face laser resurfacing can erase twenty or more years from the perceived age of a patient. The patients shown in figs. 6.3 and 6.4 were both treated only with laser resurfacing.

Because the CO_2 laser produces greater heating of the skin than does the erbium:YAG laser, resurfacing with the CO_2 laser is inherently more painful. In almost all cases, injected anesthetics are required. It is not unusual to use even general anesthesia for CO_2 laser resurfacing. For several reasons, my preference is to use local anesthesia. General anesthesia carries certain systemic risks; there's even a small but finite risk of death. Upon reversal of general anesthesia (waking up), there is no continued anesthetic effect in the

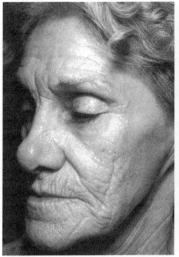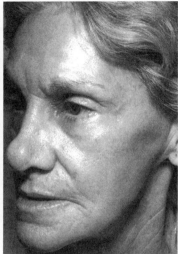

Fig. 6.4 This 63-year-old patient underwent full face laser resurfacing using the CO_2 and erbium lasers with only local anesthesia. Notice the nearly total smoothing of wrinkles, the significant tightening of cheek skin and the improvement of the nasolabial furrow (the deep fold that extends from the nose to the corner of the mouth).

treated skin area; thus longer-term anesthesia is inadequate if only general anesthesia is used.

Local anesthesia is extremely safe. Properly administered local anesthetics are 100% effective. The treated area is completely numb and the laser treatment is thus painless. Another great advantage of local anesthetics is that their effect lasts for several hours. There is generally a stinging sensation felt as the local anesthetics wear off; this pain is significantly lessened by the use of occlusive (covering) dressings over the treated skin.

I routinely perform full-face CO_2 laser resurfacing using only local anesthesia. Before anesthetics are given, pretreatment photographs are taken and major wrinkles marked with a pen. Larger areas of the face, including the forehead and the central face below the outer corners of the eyes, are efficiently numbed with nerve blocks. A nerve block is achieved by injecting a small amount of local anesthetic solution around the origin of a sensory nerve. Nerves branch out from this origin to provide sensation to a large facial area. If the nerve is blocked near its origin, the entire facial area served by the nerve becomes numb. Because some pain is associated with administering nerve blocks (as every dental patient knows!), I will usually precede these injections with a small dose of sedative medication (similar to Valium). Most patients are more comfortable if given some degree of sedation. The patients in figs. 6.3 and 6.4 received this method of anesthesia prior to laser resurfacing.

Lateral facial areas, including the temples and cheeks outside of the outer corner of the eye, also require numbing. My preference is to inject a diluted local anesthetic solution (as used for liposuction procedures) just below the skin in the fat layer of the cheek. This diluted local anesthetic solution can be injected nearly painlessly, and tends to inflate the outer cheeks due to its volume. Local anesthetics are effective over a period of several hours; the period immediately following laser resurfacing is thus completely painless.

The first two laser passes are delivered to the wrinkle shoulders (the edges of a wrinkle parallel to and on either side of the deeper trough within the wrinkle). This extra treatment adjacent to wrinkles results in superior eradication of the wrinkles. Next, with the use of a robotic scanner, large areas of the face can be resurfaced efficiently. The first pass (complete coverage of the facial area with laser energy) provides enough heating of the epidermis to enable its complete removal with a wiping action using moist cotton applicators or gauze pads. Most facial areas are treated with two additional laser passes covering the entire surface area. Because these laser passes are treating exposed dermis, which is rich in water, significant energy absorption and limited heat production occurs. This heating is sufficient to cause immediate contraction of collagen, the skin's most abundant protein, but is significantly less than would result in a thermal burn. Thus, there is no charring or carbonization of the tissue, only a rather dramatic visible tightening. The heating of the dermis is also sufficient to cause coagulation of blood vessels; thus, there is generally no bleeding during CO_2 laser resurfacing.

There is a limit to how much heat can be safely imparted to the skin by the CO_2 laser. Generally, three or four passes are the limit. Too many passes may desiccate the skin and result in excessive heat generation with subsequent laser passes. Such excessive heating can result in a burn injury with resultant scar formation or pigmentary alteration. Care must be taken to use less laser energy in certain areas of the face where the skin is thinner so that not too much of the dermis is affected. Reduced laser energy is also necessary on the eyelids because too much skin contraction of the lower eyelid can result in permanent ectropion (a pulling down of the lid that causes the white of the eye to be overly visible).

Although most wrinkles will have disappeared after three or four CO_2 laser passes, deeper wrinkles generally persist. Because additional CO_2 laser treatment may be hazardous, further resurfacing should be done using the erbium:YAG laser. Its great safety advantages allow for continued, deeper resurfacing and greater wrinkle eradication than is possible with the CO_2 laser alone. Full-face laser resurfacing ideally should be performed using both CO_2 and erbium:YAG lasers. The CO_2 laser provides the benefit of overall skin tightening, whereas the erbium:YAG laser provides the more aggressive resurfacing needed to improve even the deepest wrinkles.

After full-face resurfacing is completed, a multilayer mask-like dressing is applied to the entire face. The layers include N-terface, an extremely thin, porous polymer material (which is also used on the inner surface of Band-Aids), antibiotic ointment, gauze pads and an elastic net-like material to hold the entire dressing together. This dressing provides occlusion and also will absorb tissue fluid, which can seep to the surface of the treated skin. The local anesthetic will wear off after several hours, resulting in a stinging sensation. The occlusive covering provided by the dressing significantly lessens this painful sensation. No special care is required for the skin while the dressing is in place (generally overnight); this allows patients to simply go home and relax after the resurfacing procedure.

The day following resurfacing, the patient returns to the physician's office. The entire dressing is removed except for the N-terface layer. Over the next four or five days the resurfaced skin requires vigilant care to optimize healing. There will be a copious amount of fluid making its way to the surface. This tissue fluid is normally present in the skin and is enveloped by the waterproof outer layer of the epidermis (the stratum corneum, see chapter 2). With the epidermis removed, this fluid tends to exude onto the surface. Compresses of cool distilled water, plain or with a small amount of vinegar added, should be applied to the skin (actually to the N-terface layer) at frequent intervals, usually at least once per hour. The compress can be done with a clean wash cloth or with paper towels. After the compress, a generous amount of antibiotic ointment (usually bacitracin) should be applied to the N-terface surface. Because N-terface is not adherent, only the antibiotic ointment keeps this thin dressing layer from falling off. There are two pitfalls to self-care of the healing skin during the first several days: 1) not doing enough compresses and 2) not applying enough antibiotic ointment. A good rule of thumb is that it is virtually impossible to overdo both the frequency of the compresses and the application of the ointment. If you are debating whether to do another compress, "just do it!"

Postoperative care after laser resurfacing is designed to optimize the rate of re-epithelialization. If healing is delayed, hypertrophy (growth) of dermal tissue may occur, leading to a hypertrophic (raised) scar. Good wound care will maximize regrowth of the epidermis. Most surgeons closely monitor patients during the two weeks following full-face laser resurfacing to make sure that patients are properly caring for their healing skin.

Infection by various microorganisms is a risk to any healing skin, including that following laser resurfacing. Generally, oral antibiotics are given for seven to ten days postoperatively. Antiviral medication is also given to prevent any activation of herpes simplex, the virus that causes cold sores. A cold sore allowed to erupt may spread to cover large areas of the face because the herpes virus grows well on de-epithelialized skin. Excessive viral growth can lead to scarring if it is not treated. Occasionally patients experience infections with candida, a type of fungus. This may necessitate treatment with an oral antifungal drug.

Pain is surprisingly mild after full-face CO_2 laser resurfacing. Most of my patients report very little pain as early as one day after resurfacing. As the skin heals, there is more often a feeling of tightness (due to skin contraction), especially around the mouth area. Most patients also report itching after several days, usually correlated with regrowth of the epidermis over most of the face.

Most patients largely heal within ten days. For several days after the epidermis has re-grown, there is significant peeling of the epidermis, producing a dry appearance. This flaky skin is treated with an ointment type moisturizer (Aquaphor). The great majority of patients are able to return to work within two weeks after resurfacing. There is always redness (erythema), which has the appearance of a sunburn. This redness will fade to pink but is usually maximal about one month following surgery. By two months following surgery, the pink color will be much lighter and usually fades completely within three to four months.

Incisional Laser Surgery

A special application of the CO_2 laser is its use as a cutting or incisional instrument. This laser can be operated in a continuous wave (CW) mode, in which the laser is not pulsed but is constantly on while it is being used. If the laser energy is focused on a very small point (typically 0.1 millimeter), the beam will cut through skin or other tissues much as would a scalpel. There is one major difference, however. The CO_2 laser coagulates (denatures) the tissue due to the heat generated as water molecules absorb the laser energy. All tissue structures are coagulated, including blood vessels. The result is a bloodless incision. A regular scalpel does not cause coagulation and invariably produces copious bleeding as it cuts through skin and other tissues. The bloodless surgery possible with the CO_2 laser can be a significant advantage during any cosmetic surgery that requires incision of tissue; it is particularly well suited to blepharoplasty (eyelid lift).

Blepharoplasty

Frequently, with aging, excessive skin and/or fat accumulates around the eyelids. There are normally fat pads above and below the eyeball called orbital fat pads. These pads function as shock absorbers and cushion the eye from sudden movement or force. A connective tissue structure called the orbital septum normally prevents these fat pads from bulging forward or protruding above the skin surface. With aging, most people will experience a weakening of the orbital septum, which allows the orbital fat pads to protrude. The protrusion can be very pronounced in the lower eyelid, producing heavy bags that may cause the person to look poorly rested.

In the upper eyelids, the usual problem is excessive skin. This skin excess can be quite extensive and will result in redundant folds of skin that cover the lid itself and sometimes even the eyelashes. The excess appears to be the result of actual stretching of the skin as well as a lowering of the position of the eyebrows due to gravitational forces and the downward pull of the muscles that cause frowning. Redundant upper eyelid skin produces a tired or sad look to the eye and reduces the apparent size of the eyes. Women with excessive upper eyelid skin find it difficult to apply eye makeup because the redundant fold of skin covers the platform of eyelid skin. Additional fullness of the upper lids may be caused by bulging orbital fat pads, as often occurs in the lower lids.

The goal of blepharoplasty is to surgically remove excessive skin and fat by direct excision. Because there are abundant blood vessels in the eyelid area, a traditional (scalpel) blepharoplasty will generally cause a great deal of bruising and swelling. In contrast, when the CO_2 laser is used, blepharoplasty is generally a bloodless procedure. Any bruising is usually the result of the needle used to inject anesthetics, not the surgical cutting. The patient in fig. 6.5 is shown before and six days after CO_2 laser blepharoplasty.

In upper eyelid blepharoplasty, excessive skin is removed via an elliptical shape excision. Before any anesthesia is given, the redundant skin is carefully measured and the planned incisions are marked (for an example of these markings, see fig. 6.5). The excessive skin usually

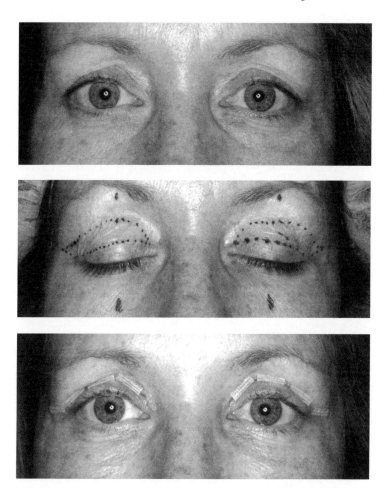

Fig. 6.5 This patient underwent CO_2 laser blepharoplasty to remove redundant skin and excessive fat in the upper eyelids. She is shown a) before surgery, b) with marking for planned removal of skin, and c) six days after blepharoplasty, with stitches removed and SteriStrips placed over the incision line. Notice that the skin removal extends slightly onto the temple and that there is minimal swelling or bruising six days later.

extends laterally to the outer corner of the eye and the skin excision must include this lateral skin. The size and shape of this skin excision is the most important factor that determines the aesthetic quality of the surgical result. After the skin surface is marked, the eyelids are numbed with a local anesthetic injection. Special eye shields, much like contact lenses, are placed directly on the eye surface after it has been numbed with anesthetic eye drops. Next, the focused CO_2 laser is used to slice through the eyelid skin. Some of the superficial herniated orbital fat is removed by slicing off fragments using the laser. The opening in the skin is stitched together to re-approximate the skin edges. Ice packs are applied for several hours after the surgery to chill the skin, constricting blood vessels and reducing swelling.

Stitches are removed by the seventh postoperative day (fig. 6.5). With proper technique there is a minimal scar along the suture line. Because upper eyelid skin heals extremely well, this scar should be virtually undetectable to the casual observer (fig. 6.6).

In the lower eyelids, the primary problem that occurs with aging is bulging of the orbital fat pads as opposed to the presence of excessive skin. In lower lid blepharoplasty, the herniated, superficial portions of the fat pads are removed. Excessive skin, if present, is best removed by laser resurfacing, which results in contraction of this skin. Using a focused CO_2 laser instead of a scalpel for blepharoplasty offers the significant advantage of bloodless surgery, affording the surgeon better visualization of important anatomic structures.

The safest approach to lower lid blepharoplasty is to access the fat pads through an incision of the conjunctiva (inner lining) of the lower lid, rather than through the skin. This transconjunctival approach has two major advantages over the skin approach. Because the fat pads lie behind the orbital septum (connective tissue layer), this septum must be traversed if the skin approach is used. Unfortunately, the orbital septum frequently heals by contracting excessively, possibly resulting in a permanent pulling down of the lower eyelid. Such pulling down can cause an unnatural shape to the eye or may reveal the white of the eye below the iris, also an unnatural appearance. With the transconjunctival technique, the fat

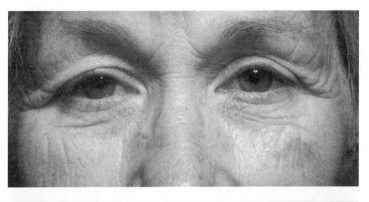

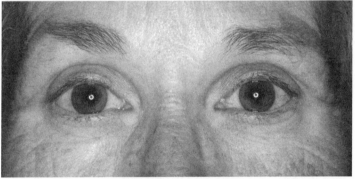

Fig. 6.6 This 60-year-old patient is shown before and after CO_2 laser blepharoplasty. Note the excessive upper eyelid skin and fat tissue in the preoperative photograph. In the postoperative photograph, note the considerably more "open eyed" look as well as the inconspicuous scar from the skin excision.

pads are accessed without traversing the orbital septum, thus avoiding the potential problem of contraction of the septum.

The other advantage of the transconjunctival technique for lower lid blepharoplasty is that it avoids a skin incision, which may heal with an observable scar. Compared to upper lid incisions, lower lid skin is more likely to scar when it heals. The transconjunctival approach totally prevents this possibility. Because the biggest risk of blepharoplasty is postoperative bleeding around the eye, the CO_2 laser method is much safer than traditional non-laser techniques.

7. Complementary Procedures to Cosmetic Laser Surgery

Many cosmetic laser surgery procedures are used in conjunction with non-laser cosmetic procedures because the effect of two or more procedures may be significantly greater than the effect of a single procedure. Different procedures frequently work through entirely different mechanisms. Taking advantage of different mechanisms of improvement can achieve optimal results. Some complementary procedures can be done at the same time; others ideally should be done in sequence, with one preceding the other by several weeks or months.

Procedures Done in Advance of Laser Resurfacing

There are several procedures, both surgical and nonsurgical, that complement laser resurfacing. Most of these complementary procedures can be performed either before or after the resurfacing, but I generally prefer to do them prior to resurfacing.

For patients with extensive sun damage, full-face resurfacing with the CO_2 laser is perhaps the single cosmetic surgery that can result in the greatest overall facial rejuvenation (see chapter 6 and figs. 6.3 and 6.4). The tightening of facial skin that results from this procedure can even afford some improvement in the loose skin of the neck. (The neck itself can also be resurfaced, but neck skin heals more slowly and is at significantly increased risk of scarring if resurfaced.) The majority of patients who are candidates for full-face laser resurfacing are middle-aged or older and have significant cosmetic problems in the neck area. Frequently there is excessive fat in the anterior neck below the chin, sometimes resulting in a double chin. Most patients will also have a prominence of the lower cheek (jowl) area, also due to excessive fat. The neck and jowls usually sag because of stretching of both the skin and the underlying fascia. With advanced sagging of these tissue layers the neck will have a "turkey gobbler" look. Some people have prominent bands running along the vertical axis of the neck, caused by a redundancy of a superficial muscle (the platysma muscle).

Most patients with cosmetic problems in the neck area require liposuction for rejuvenation of this area. I usually perform liposuction of both neck and jowl areas, because most patients have excessive fatty tissue in both. Those patients who have relatively little sagging of the lower cheeks and neck but who have excess fat in these areas may require only liposuction. Those who have significant sagging will generally also need to have a facelift procedure (see below). I perform both of these procedures using the tumescent technique of local anesthesia. With this method, the subcutaneous tissue (the fat layer) is diffusely infiltrated with a dilute solution of local anesthetic in saline (salt water). The solution contains the anesthetic lidocaine, which completely numbs the area, and epinephrine, which causes significant constriction of the blood vessels. Tumescent local anesthesia has several major advantages. It is extremely safe, because the effects of the anesthesia are confined to the local area of infiltration, and there are no systemic effects from these drugs. Because the local blood vessels are constricted, there is minimal bleeding during surgery and thus very little postoperative bruising and swelling. Recovery from surgery is very rapid because of the minimal bruising and swelling.

Liposuction of the neck and jowls and facelift are conveniently performed simultaneously and generally prior (one month or more) to full-face laser resurfacing. These procedures cannot be done simultaneously with laser resurfacing because, after liposuction and/ or facelift, a chin strap–style compression garment, which covers much of the cheek area, must be worn for a few days. This garment

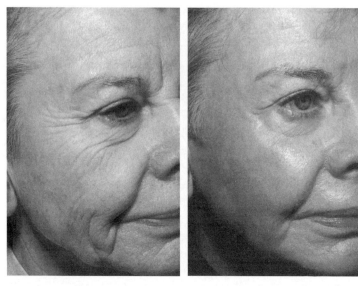

Fig. 7.1 This 74-year-old patient had prominent fat in the neck and jowls (lower cheek) areas and underwent liposuction of these areas. She subsequently received full face laser resurfacing.

would interfere with the postoperative care needed after laser resurfacing. Recovery after liposuction of the neck and jowls and/or facelift is very rapid, with most patients able to resume normal activities, including work, within one week of surgery. The patient in fig. 7.1 underwent liposuction of the neck and jowls, followed 12 months later by full-face laser resurfacing.

In most patients with redundant platysma muscle, I perform a corset platysmaplasty procedure along with liposuction of neck and jowls. This procedure is essentially a "facelift for the neck" because the platysma muscle layer is continuous with the fascia on the face that is tightened during a facelift. The only anesthesia needed for platysmaplasty is the same local (tumescent) anesthesia that is used for liposuction. Immediately after liposuction of the neck and jowls, a small horizontal skin incision is made in the transverse crease that lies just below the chin. Through this incision, scissors are used to separate the skin from the underlying flat platysma muscle. The edges of the left and right platysma muscles are stitched together with a continuous suture, much like an old-fashioned corset. Stitching together the muscle edges provides tightening of this layer and is very effective at smoothing the neck and eliminating the platysma bands.

Many patients with excessive laxity of the lower face and neck tissues benefit from a facelifting procedure. A newer technique, developed in Europe, is the S-lift minimum incision facelift. I frequently use this technique in combination with liposuction of the neck and jowls, with or without corset platysmaplasty, using entirely local tumescent anesthesia. The S-lift technique is analogous to the platysmaplasty in the neck, in that the goal is to tighten the fascia (SMAS) layer. In the S-lift small skin incisions (shaped like the letter *S*) are made in front of each ear; next, a dissection is made in the fatty layer just beneath the skin of the lateral cheek and lateral neck. The fascia layer is then pulled in an upward direction from the lateral neck toward the ear and is anchored to the periosteum (a tough connective tissue layer) of a bone in front of the ear, using permanent suture material. Another stitch is used to tighten the SMAS layer of the cheek, pulling it up and sideways toward the ear. A small amount of excess cheek skin is excised and the skin is then stitched together.

I have found that the S-lift minimum incision facelift results in remarkable improvement and achieves most of the results of a standard facelift. Compared to conventional facelift surgery, this mini-facelift has several advantages. One is that this procedure can be done entirely with local anesthesia. Other advantages include minimal bruising and swelling and a very rapid recovery, usually in only a few days. (In fact, some of my patients have returned to work three days after the S-lift procedure.) With the S-lift, surgery is limited to safe areas of the face, virtually eliminating the risk of damage to nerves or blood vessels that is associated with traditional facelifts. Another advantage of the S-lift is that the only visible part of the skin incision is immediately in front of the ear, generally within a natural crease and thus inconspicuous. In contrast, the traditional facelift produces a much larger and longer scar that extends onto the neck and scalp behind the ear.

The combination of liposuction of neck and jowls and/or S-lift minimum incision facelift followed by full-face laser resurfacing can result in complete rejuvenation of the mid-to-lower face and neck areas entirely through minimally invasive procedures using only local anesthesia.

Another procedure that would ideally precede full-face laser resurfacing and is sometimes performed in conjunction with a lower eyelid blepharoplasty is the lateral canthal tendon suspension. This procedure is done in those patients who have excessively lax lower eyelids and who are at risk of developing, or may already have, ectropion, a condition in which the lower eyelid is excessively loose and may even be chronically separated from contact with the surface of the eye. This procedure is well suited to a focused CO_2 laser technique and can also be performed using only local anesthesia. An incision is made in the temple area near where the upper and lower eyelids come together, and the tendon that runs along the lower eyelid margin is anchored to the fibrous tissue just above the bony layer. Because the CO_2 laser is used, this procedure is bloodless and produces less swelling and faster healing than that experienced with conventional scalpel surgery.

Botox Injection: A Nonsurgical Method for Reducing Facial Wrinkles

Botulinum toxin (Botox) is a medication with the unique property of relaxing muscles after direct injection into the muscle. This medication is a purified protein produced by *clostridium botulinum*, the bacterium that causes botulism. Botulism occurs in humans when they are exposed to large doses of botulinum toxin, usually by ingesting food that has been contaminated with the bacterium. The disease can be fatal if large amounts of the toxin are ingested because the toxin causes paralysis of all muscles, including those required for breathing. Extremely small doses of botulinum toxin are effective at safely paralyzing the muscles into which it is injected (without producing any systemic effect because it does not reach other parts of the body). The paralysis produced by Botox injection is temporary (3–6 month duration).

At the nerve ending between motor nerve cells and skeletal muscle cells, molecules of the neurotransmitter acetylcholine are released from the nerve cell and migrate to the muscle cell where they attach to a surface receptor and activate muscle contraction. Botulinum toxin enters the nerve cells and destroys proteins that are needed for the release of acetylcholine. The toxin permanently disables the nerve endings and the muscle cell becomes paralyzed. Over the next few months, however, new, normally functioning nerve endings grow from the nerve cell, eventually restoring the cell's ability to release acetylcholine and stimulate muscle contraction. The muscle will then function normally until the next injection of Botox.

Most facial wrinkles occur as a result of repeated contraction of muscles of expression (fig. 2.4). Botox injection will produce significant improvement in wrinkles and furrows, partly because opposing muscles that have not been treated tend to pull the skin in a direction that actively smoothes the wrinkles during the months that Botox is active.

Botox was first approved by the FDA in 1989 as a treatment for spastic eye and neck muscles. In 2002, it was approved for cosmetic use to relax the small muscles that cause frowning. Studies are under way for non-cosmetic uses of Botox, including treating migraine headaches, inhibiting excess sweating, relaxing spastic urinary bladder (a common cause of incontinence), and even treating obesity by relaxing the muscles of the stomach wall to slow gastric emptying.

Botox is administered by injection with a small needle directly into the muscles to be treated. The most common side effect is bruising from the needle. Another risk is unintended paralysis of nearby muscles because of diversion of the toxin from the site of injection. The most common example of this problem is drooping of the eyelid after injection of frown muscles. Patients who are pregnant or nursing should not receive Botox, not should patients with myasthenia gravis, a neurological disease that may be worsened by treatment.

In 1995, while attending a medical seminar, I received my first injection of Botox into my frown line area. I was impressed with the improvement in my rather pronounced frown lines. A few weeks later I visited a cosmetic laser surgeon. It occurred to me that undergoing laser resurfacing of my frown line area might produce superior results because these muscles were paralyzed, and the healing skin would not be subject to the folding forces that occur with each frown. In July 1995 I had my frown line area treated by CO_2 laser resurfacing. To my knowledge, I was the first patient to undergo laser resurfacing while under the influence of Botox. Since then, I have given myself Botox treatments every few months in the frown line area. As of 2004 (nine years later) there has been no recurrence of any wrinkling in this area.

The theory behind combining Botox treatment with laser resurfacing is that the healing skin is not subject to wrinkling because the muscles are relaxed. As new layers of skin are regenerated, the newly synthesized collagen fibers are randomly distributed and thus more resistant to the recurrence of wrinkles even after the Botox effect has worn off. This concept has been verified by analysis of wrinkle recurrence, which was found to be delayed after combined Botox/laser resurfacing treatment.

Reducing Facial Scars

As discussed in chapter 6, resurfacing with the erbium:YAG laser is a very effective treatment for facial scars. Resurfacing is most effective for small diameter, superficial scars. Large-diameter, deeper scars require adjunctive treatments that result in elevation of the scar or thickening of the depressed skin within the scar. One such treatment is subcision, a minor surgical procedure done under local anesthesia. In this process, a hypodermic needle is used as a small surgical scalpel to slice through scar tissue bands below the type III scar. Releasing the scar tissue allows the "bound down" skin to elevate. The injury produced by subcision heals with the production of additional dermal tissue (collagen), which also contributes to thickening of the skin within the depressed scar, thus elevating the depression. Because the skin surface is essentially undisturbed by subcision, these treatments produce little immediately noticeable effect other than minor bruising or swelling. All the healing takes place beneath the skin surface. These treatments can be done anytime before or after laser resurfacing.

Another method of elevating type III depressed scars is injection of a filler material. Bovine collagen is widely used for this purpose. I prefer injecting Fascian to provide filling. Fascian is composed mainly of human collagen derived from fascia obtained from tissue donors. Unlike bovine collagen, there is virtually no risk of an allergic reaction from human collagen. The human material also persists longer after injection—generally six months, compared to three months for bovine collagen.

Small-diameter, deep acne scars are not amenable to laser resurfacing. These scars are classified as type II acne scars and are sometimes called "ice pick" scars because of their shape. Type II acne scars are best treated by total removal, usually done with a small, round punch biopsy instrument using local anesthesia (fig. 6.2). The punch instrument removes a small cylinder of skin, including the entire scar. If the removed scars are small, the remaining normal skin is simply stitched together. Larger scars leave a larger punch defect and may require filling with a small skin graft, which is also obtained with the punch biopsy instrument, usually from skin behind the ear (of the same patient). Punch removal of type II acne scars is usually performed several weeks prior to laser resurfacing.

Non-Ablative Laser Treatments to Improve Wrinkles

Laser resurfacing is the most reliable method for smoothing facial wrinkles. During resurfacing, skin tissue is ablated layer by layer. A healing period always follows resurfacing, during which superficial skin layers grow back to replace the layers that were removed. The major landmark of healing is re-epithelialization.

In 1998, an alternative laser treatment designed to improve facial wrinkles without ablating the epidermis was introduced. This method, called CoolTouch, uses a special Nd:YAG laser with a wavelength of 1320 nm. This long wavelength penetrates deep into the dermis and is relatively invisible to the epidermis. The energy passes through the epidermis and its effect is confined to the dermis, where it is absorbed by water, thus generating heat. The small amount of heat generated in the dermis appears to produce a minor injury, which in turn may stimulate the fibroblast cells to produce new collagen. Clinical studies in which skin biopsies were examined have revealed the synthesis of new collagen as a result of CoolTouch treatment and visible improvement in facial wrinkles.

The main advantage of CoolTouch treatment is the avoidance of an obvious healing process and thus no down time for treated patients. Disadvantages include the need for multiple treatments, variable results experienced by different patients, and rather modest improvement in wrinkles. The degree of improvement is generally significantly less than that achieved by laser resurfacing.

A similar non-ablative laser treatment is performed with the Q-switched Nd:YAG laser operating at 1064 nm. This wavelength also has a negligible effect on the epidermis and affects primarily the dermis. When used at higher fluences (above those used to treat tattoos), these treatments may result in purpura but will not significantly affect the epidermis. Similar to results from CoolTouch treatments, modest improvement in facial wrinkles usually occurs after a series of treatments with the Q-switched Nd:YAG laser.

Two additional non-ablative resurfacing modalities are the pulsed dye laser and an intense pulsed light (IPL) source. The same pulsed dye laser as that used for treating vascular lesions (see chapter 4), as well as a newer version that has a longer pulse duration, have been used for this purpose. Although the short wavelength of the pulsed dye laser does not penetrate very deeply into the dermis, physicians have noticed serendipitous improvement of both fine wrinkles and skin texture in patients who have received multiple treatments for facial telangiectases. The wavelength of light produced by the pulsed dye laser is well absorbed by both hemoglobin and melanin. Improvement in skin texture is thought to be the result of nonspecific heating of water in the superficial dermis, secondary to heating of the primary pigmented tissue. A slight injury is produced, stimulating fibroblasts in the dermis to produce more collagen.

The IPL source is not a laser; it is a flashlamp that produces non-coherent light over a broad spectrum of visible and infrared wavelengths. Filters are used to eliminate part of the output spectrum. Response of the skin to this intense light is similar in many respects to its response to laser energy of similar wavelength, power, and pulse duration. The most common IPL source is the Photoderm, which is generally used to treat vascular and pigmented lesions using wavelengths in the 500–800 nm range. When used on the face, subtle improvement in skin texture and fine wrinkles has been noted, similar to that observed following non-ablative laser treatment. Filters can also be used that allow delivery of infrared wavelengths up to 1200 nm. This infrared energy has less effect on pigmented targets and will produce greater heating of water, resulting in increased collagen synthesis and improved skin texture.

Recently, additional lasers have been developed for non-ablative skin texture improvement. These include a diode laser operating at 1450 nm ("Smoothbeam") and an erbium:glass laser operating at 1540 nm. Both of these wavelengths are absorbed mainly by water and can improve skin texture, but have little effect on excess melanin or hemoglobin pigments.

Non-Laser Devices for Facial Resurfacing

Microdermabrasion is a noninvasive resurfacing modality used to gently remove only the superficial layer of the epidermis (the stratum corneum, see chapter 2). First developed in Europe, these treatments were introduced in the United States in the late 1990s and have gained great popularity. The chief appeal of microdermabrasion is that multiple treatments can improve skin texture and lessen the appearance of fine wrinkles and even acne scars, all with no detectable healing response or down time for patients. With standard techniques, there is minimal facial redness for only several hours following treatment.

Microdermabrasion works in a method reminiscent of sandblasting, by gently blowing tiny aluminum oxide crystals at high velocity against the skin surface. Repeated passes over the treated area can result in deeper levels of epidermal ablation, but such aggressive abrasion would defeat the goal of a minimally invasive treatment. Clinical studies that include skin biopsy samples have demonstrated increased collagen production in the dermis as well as thickening of the viable epidermal cell layers as a result of a series of microdermabrasion treatments. It is remarkable that microscopic changes were evident in the dermis, because the immediate effect of these treatments is confined to superficial layers of the epidermis. Presumably, epidermal cells are able to convey a biochemical signal to dermal cells that results in increased collagen production.

Compared to non-ablative laser treatments, microdermabrasion may more quickly result in visible improvement. In addition to its non-ablative nature and its effect on dermal collagen, and unlike non-ablative laser treatments, microdermabrasion directly smoothes the superficial epidermis and provides rapid improvement in skin texture. This improved texture is a benefit that patients immediately appreciate.

Another newer treatment is Coblation. The name is derived from "cold ablation" because this apparatus removes skin layers without significant heat generation. This is a novel electrosurgical modality in which an electrical current creates a plasma (a type of "melting" of the tissue) on the skin surface, destroying the tissue and enabling its removal layer by layer. Multiple passes over the skin using Coblation will remove skin as far down as the dermal layer. The electrical current also coagulates blood vessels, resulting in bloodless skin removal.

Coblation is clearly an ablative modality and necessitates healing via re-epithelialization. This method is most similar to laser resurfacing with the erbium:YAG laser. Both treatments are ablative and generate insignificant heating of the skin. One disadvantage of

Coblation is that the treatment head is a fixed size and thus requires that a swath of skin of this width be treated. In contrast, the erbium:YAG laser employs various spot sizes, some less than 2 mm wide, enabling greater precision of skin removal. Skin surface features such as wrinkle shoulders and acne scars can be selectively ablated with the erbium:YAG laser.

8. Getting Good Results

High-quality results are attributable much more to the surgeon than to the laser. Although any physician who follows a rote "cookbook" approach to laser surgery can achieve results, outstanding results require significant skill on the part of the surgeon. Top-quality laser surgeons usually develop their own techniques. Surgeons who perform many laser procedures constantly refine their technique and are able to achieve substantial improvement for the patient while avoiding the risks associated with over-treatment.

One of the strongest indicators of the commitment and skills of laser surgeons is whether they possess their own laser equipment. Lasers are very expensive machines and for economic reasons will not be acquired by a physician who has only a casual interest in using them. Many laser rental companies will bring a laser into a physician's office on a per case or per diem basis. A physician who rents a laser once a month is clearly not dealing with many laser surgery cases and in all probability lacks sufficient experience to achieve optimal results. Surgeons who use a laser only in a hospital or outpatient surgery center are also less likely to have a great deal of experience. It is a very good sign that you are dealing with an experienced laser surgeon if the surgeon owns the equipment and uses it in his or her office.

How do you find the best surgeon? By far the best way is through word of mouth. The recommendation of a trusted friend or family member is an excellent indicator of the surgeon's quality. An impartial physician such as your primary care provider may also be able to recommend a laser cosmetic surgeon in whom they have confidence. Any surgeon can pay to advertise or gain recognition in the media through a public relations agent. The surgeon you have heard a lot about in the media may not be the best one in your area.

What about the medical specialty of the laser surgeon? Dermatologists are the ultimate skin care experts and dominate the field of cosmetic laser surgery. Because they are most familiar with the skin, dermatologists are the surgeons least likely to experience complications with surgery or healing and are also the best qualified to prevent, recognize, and treat complications before they become a significant problem. There are also many highly qualified laser surgeons from the fields of general plastic surgery (also called plastic and reconstructive surgery), facial plastic surgery (trained primarily as ear, nose and throat surgeons), and oculoplastic surgery (trained primarily as ophthalmologists or eye surgeons).

Another excellent indicator of cosmetic laser surgeons' skills and abilities are their professional activities in this field. Active surgeons are innovators who develop improved surgical techniques, present their results at national and international meetings of surgical societies, and publish their findings in peer reviewed medical journals. (Peer review is an anonymous editorial process in which expert physicians in the field criticize an article submitted for publication and may reject it for publication if it does not meet scientific standards of quality.) Some of the most important professional societies and their respective scientific journals include the American Society for Dermatologic Surgery (*Dermatologic Surgery*), the American Academy of Facial Plastic Surgery (*Archives of Facial Plastic Surgery*), the American Society for Lasers in Medicine and Surgery (*Lasers in Surgery and Medicine*), the American Society of Plastic Surgeons (*Plastic and Reconstructive Surgery*), and the International Society of Cosmetic Laser Surgeons (*Dermatologic Surgery*).

When you visit a physician's office for a consultation on cosmetic laser surgery, the surgeon may recommend one or more procedures. The surgeon should explain to you why a given procedure is a good choice for you and why it is preferred over alternative treatments. You should be shown photographs of the surgeon's actual patients who have received the proposed surgery. (You may also ask to contact some of these patients to inquire about their experience with laser surgery.) You should be informed of what to expect before and after the surgery, what happens during the procedure, what the recovery will be like, and the potential risks and complications. It is your responsibility to reveal your complete relevant medical history including any allergies, bleeding problems, abnormal healing or tendencies to scar after surgery, and problems with infections (especially cold sores, or herpes virus infections).

Your expectations for laser or other cosmetic surgery must be realistic, or you may find yourself disappointed with the results of surgery. How do you know if your expectations are realistic? One of the most important tasks of the surgeon is to make sure that they are. During the consultation, the surgeon should have you look into a mirror and describe exactly what facial features you would like to improve. The surgeon then should be able to tell you what a recommended surgical procedure would likely accomplish. Sometimes, optimal results may require a combination of two or more procedures. Looking at photographs of previous patients who have undergone the same procedures can be helpful in clarifying your expectations for surgery. Experienced surgeons are strongly motivated to make sure that their cosmetic surgery patients have realistic expectations. The last thing they want is a disappointed patient.

As you contemplate undergoing laser or any type of cosmetic surgery, you should ask yourself what your motivations are. This is a personal decision and should be taken to meet your expectations, not those of others. If you are truly concerned about some aspect of your appearance and would like to see it improved, you should certainly consider cosmetic surgery. If your expectations of the surgery are met or exceeded, you will likely be pleased with your results and will know that you made the right decision.

Advances in cosmetic laser surgery have made possible the safe removal of a wide variety of skin imperfections including excess hair, enlarged blood vessels, and pigmented lesions. Laser resurfacing, although a more invasive surgical procedure, can produce remarkable improvement in wrinkled and sun damaged skin. (In fact, the more wrinkled and sun damaged the skin, the more dramatic will be the likely improvement.) Incisional laser surgery, especially blepharoplasty, produces the same results as conventional surgery, only with much less bruising and a much faster recovery. The laser is not a magic wand, but in the hands of a skilled surgeon this instrument can produce remarkable cosmetic improvement.

Glossary

These terms are defined in a way that is specific to the field of cosmetic laser surgery, and may have different or broader meanings in other contexts.

Ablation Removal of tissue, usually by a pulsed surgical laser (for example, erbium:YAG or CO_2) that vaporizes the water contained in the tissue. Ablation causes minimal damage to adjacent non-ablated tissue (in contrast to *coagulation*).

Basal layer Lowermost (innermost) layer of the *epidermis*, adjacent to the *dermis*. Location of basal *keratinocytes* and *melanocytes*.

Blepharoplasty Surgical removal of excessive skin and/or fatty tissue from the eyelids.

Botox (trademark) An FDA-approved preparation of *botulinum toxin* used to temporarily relax muscles that cause facial wrinkles, such as frown lines.

Botulinum toxin A protein produced by the bacterium *Clostridia botulinum*. The toxin binds to nerve endings and prevents the motor nerve stimulus from activating muscle contraction, thus temporarily paralyzing the muscle.

Capillaries The smallest blood vessels. Capillaries are present throughout the *dermis* but are not present in the *epidermis*.

Chromophore A molecule or entity that selectively absorbs laser energy of a specific wavelength. For example, the *hemoglobin* chromophore selectively absorbs the energy output of the pulsed dye laser, and the water chromophore absorbs the energy output of the erbium:YAG laser.

Coagulation A type of damage to tissue caused by very high temperatures, for example that generated by a continuous-wave CO_2 laser. The heat denatures tissue proteins and can seal blood vessels during surgery, thus minimizing bleeding.

Coblation Skin resurfacing surgery in which an electrosurgical instrument removes layers of skin by *ablation*. A non-laser treatment analogous to erbium:YAG *laser resurfacing*.

Coherence A property of laser energy that describes the fact that light waves of laser energy are in synchrony with each other. The peaks and troughs of the light waves are perfectly in line.

Collagen The major component of the *dermis*. Collagen fibers are inelastic and provide the skin's strength.

Collimation A property of laser energy that describes the fact that light waves of laser energy are parallel to each other.

CoolTouch (trademark) An infrared laser used for non-ablative facial rejuvenation.

Dermis Layer of the skin beneath the *epidermis*. The dermis varies widely in thickness in different parts of the body and is composed mostly of extracellular material including proteins and water. The major proteins of the dermis include *collagen* and elastin (elastic fibers). The predominant cells in the dermis are *fibroblasts* (the cells that produce collagen and elastic fibers). The dermis also includes blood and lymph vessels, glands, hair follicles, and nerves.

Differentiation A complex maturation process in which newly produced cells undergo transformation into a more specialized cell type. Best illustrated in the *epidermis*, in which *keratinocytes* multiply in the innermost *basal layer* (where they are small and round) and progressively differentiate into the large flat (dead) cells that compose the outermost *stratum corneum*. The cells demonstrate obvious changes in appearance as they progress through the intervening *prickle cell layer* and *granular cell layer*.

Electromagnetic spectrum The full range of electromagnetic energy from very high energy (short wavelength) gamma rays to very low energy (long wavelength) radio waves. Visible light ranges from 400 nm (violet) to 700 nm (red) wavelength. Shorter wavelengths are referred to as *ultraviolet*, longer wavelengths are called *infrared*.

Electron Subatomic particle that orbits the nucleus of an atom. The electron carries a negative charge and will occupy specific orbits determined by its energy level.

Epidermis Outer layers of the skin comprising a dead portion and an inner living portion. Contains several layers of *keratinocytes* in varying levels of *differentiation,* and provides a physical barrier with the environment outside the body. Also includes *melanocytes* (pigment-producing cells).

Fascia A tough connective tissue layer (composed mainly of collagen) that covers many muscles in the body and provides a physical connection between muscles and more superficial structures. The superficial fascia of the face (*SMAS*) is attached to the skin via connective tissue. When the facial muscles contract, the fascia conveys facial expression to the skin.

Fibroblast The major cell type in the *dermis.* Fibroblasts produce the protein molecules that assemble into *collagen* and elastic fibers. These fibers provide both strength and elasticity to the skin.

Flashlamp An intensely bright electric lamp that flashes on for a very brief period. Used in certain types of lasers as an energy source to stimulate the excitable molecules within the laser chamber.

Granular cell layer Epidermal layer just above the *prickle cell layer.* *Keratinocytes* of this layer are more highly differentiated than in lower layers and exhibit dark color granules when viewed with a microscope.

Hemangioma A type of benign tumor, composed of blood vessels (mainly *capillaries*), that arises in the *dermis.* A hemangioma will appear as a red lesion and is usually elevated above the surrounding skin. Many hemangiomas appear in early childhood and if not treated will grow for several months, then shrink and largely disappear, leaving an area of scar tissue in the skin.

Hemoglobin The red, iron-containing protein within red blood cells that binds oxygen molecules for transport from the lungs to the tissues of the body.

Hemosiderin A brown or orange pigment that appears in the skin after red blood cells have leaked out of blood vessels into the *dermis.* Hemosiderin results from the breakdown of *hemoglobin* and has a large iron component.

Incisional surgery A type of surgery in which tissue is cut out (incised) as with a scalpel blade or a focused CO_2 laser.

Infrared Electromagnetic energy with wavelengths longer than 700 *nanometers*. Beyond the visible light spectrum, with energy levels lower than those of red light (infra = below).

Keratinocyte The predominant cell type of the *epidermis*. These cells produce a protein called keratin.

Laser An acronym for Light Amplification by the Stimulated Emission of Radiation. This term is used to describe the physical process by which laser energy is produced as well as the machine (a laser) that produces laser energy.

Laser resurfacing A surgical procedure in which an ablative (see *ablation*) laser is used to remove superficial layers of skin.

Lentigo See *solar lentigo*.

Liposuction Surgical procedure in which *subcutaneous* fat is removed via suction. Usually done with *tumescent anesthesia* (tumescent liposuction).

Macrophage A relatively large white blood cell that migrates from *capillaries* to other tissues, including the *dermis*. These cells ingest debris (including tattoo ink particles) and remove it from the skin by migrating into lymphatic vessels and transporting the debris to nearby lymph nodes or to the liver.

Melanin Proteinaceous pigment in skin that screens out ultraviolet light.

Melanocyte Melanin-producing cell in the *epidermis*.

Melanosome The organelle (membrane-bound structure) within the melanocyte that synthesizes *melanin*. Melanin gets into *keratinocytes* by the transfer of melanosomes.

Microdermabrasion A mild facial treatment in which tiny particles (usually aluminum oxide) are blown against the skin at high velocity, gently "sandblasting" superficial epidermal layers.

Monochromicity The property of being composed of a single wavelength of electromagnetic radiation (for example, a single color of light in the visible spectrum) (mono = one, chroma = color). A feature of laser energy.

Nanometer One billionth of a meter. Abbreviated as nm.

Nanosecond One billionth of a second . Abbreviated as nsec.

Nevus (pl. **nevi**) A skin lesion composed of cells that are normally present in the skin but that are increased in number. There are several types of nevi; they are denoted by the type of skin cell involved. A melanocytic nevus is composed of increased numbers of *melanocytes*. An epidermal nevus is composed of increased numbers of *keratinocytes*.

Orbicularis oris A circular muscle that surrounds the mouth. When this muscle contracts, the lips pucker.

Photon The fundamental unit of electromagnetic energy. The photon has properties of both a particle and a wave.

Platysma A broad, thin muscle that attaches to the clavicle (collarbone) and runs up the side of the neck and onto the cheeks, where it is continuous with the *SMAS fascia*.

Port wine stain A common birthmark composed of a flat red patch of skin. In a port wine stain, the *capillaries* in the *dermis* are chronically dilated. If untreated, with age a port wine stain may become darker and develop raised components.

Prickle cell layer Epidermal layer just above the *basal layer*. In the prickle cell layer the *keratinocytes* are larger than in the *basal layer* and exhibit spiny attachments to each other.

Q-switched laser A laser with an extremely short pulse (5–40 *nanoseconds*). Used for nonsurgical removal of tattoo ink or skin pigment.

Quantum theory The theory that radiant energy is composed of finite quanta; explains the structure of atoms and molecules and how energy and matter interact.

Selective photothermolysis The underlying principle of cosmetic laser treatments. Light (photo) of a specific wavelength is selectively absorbed by a targeted *chromophore* in the skin, generating enough heat (thermo) to destroy (lyse) the tissue. The effect of the laser is selective because the unwanted skin component (the chromophore) readily absorbs laser energy of the chosen wavelength. Skin components other than the chromophore are not affected.

SMAS Superficial musculo-aponeurotic system: the superficial muscles of the face along with the *fascia* that connects them. The SMAS includes the *platysma* muscle on the lower cheek and neck. In a facelift operation, the SMAS is pulled upwards and backwards (usually with sutures) to reverse the sagging that occurs with aging.

Solar elastosis Changes in the skin caused by chronic sun exposure. A sign of photo-aging that includes increased amounts of abnormal elastic fibers in the *dermis.*

Solar keratosis A skin lesion caused by chronic exposure to sunlight. Also referred to as actinic keratoses (plural), these lesions appear as rough red patches in the most sun-exposed areas of the body, especially the face. Most solar keratoses are one-quarter inch or less in diameter. If not treated they may progress to become a squamous cell carcinoma (skin cancer).

Solar lentigo A flat, brown spot that appears in areas of the skin chronically exposed to sunlight. Similar to a freckle, these age spots are patches of skin that contain increased amounts of *melanin,* the skin pigment.

Stratum corneum Topmost (outer) epidermal layer. Composed of terminally differentiated *keratinocytes* that have died and become large and flat. The stratum corneum functions as a protective barrier with the outside environment and also prevents water loss from lower skin layers. The dead cells of the stratum corneum flake off as they are replaced by new cells from below.

Subcision A minor surgical procedure in which the sharp edge of a hypodermic needle is used to cut through connective tissue and scar tissue. Used to help elevate depressed scars.

Subcutaneous Beneath the skin.

Telangiectasia A visibly dilated blood vessel, generally less than 1mm in diameter. May appear on the face as a result of chronic sun damage or in association with rosacea (an acne-like skin disease).

Tumescent anesthesia A method of local anesthesia used for surgery in which a relatively dilute local anesthetic drug, usually lidocaine (dissolved in a salt-water solution) is injected into tissue. A relatively large volume of the anesthetic solution is injected to ensure that the tissue is completely anesthetized. The tumescent anesthetic solution usually includes a low concentration of epinephrine, a drug that causes blood vessels to constrict (greatly reducing bleeding during surgery).

Ultraviolet Electromagnetic energy situated beyond the violet end of the visible spectrum (ultra = beyond); wavelengths are shorter than 400 *nanometers.*

Index

Understanding Health and Sickness Series
Miriam Bloom, Ph.D., General Editor

Also in this series

Addiction • Alzheimer's Disease • Anemia • Asthma • Breast Cancer
Genetics • Childhood Obesity • Chronic Pain • Colon Cancer •
Crohn Disease and Ulcerative Colitis • Cystic Fibrosis • Dental Health
• Depression • Hepatitis • Herpes • Mental Retardation • Migraine
and Other Headaches • Panic and Other Anxiety Disorders • Sickle
Cell Disease • Stuttering